Special Project Report

Expanding the Medicaid Program in Texas: Funding Issues and Alternatives

A report by Anne Dunkelberg
Lyndon B. Johnson School of Public Affairs
The University of Texas at Austin

1988

Anne Dunkelberg is a Research Analyst for the Texas Research League. A graduate of The University of Texas at Austin, she received a Bachelor of Arts degree in the Plan II Interdisciplinary Program in 1979 and a master's degree in 1988 from the Lyndon B. Johnson School of Public Affairs. As part of her master's degree requirement, she served an internship at the Texas Research League in Austin, Texas, and prepared this Professional Report.

ISBN: 0-89940-861-3
Library of Congress Catalog Card No.: 88-82332

Printed in the U.S.A.

This report is dedicated to the memory of
my mother, Carolyn Harris Dunkelberg.

ACKNOWLEDGEMENTS

I would like to thank Professor David C. Warner for his invaluable and enthusiastic guidance in this project, and Professor Lynn F. Anderson for agreeing to be my second reader. Thanks must also go to the Texas Research League for their patient support, and to the many people at the Texas Department of Human Services and the Texas Department of Health who assisted me in my research.

Anne Dunkelberg

The University of Texas at Austin
August, 1988

Table of Contents

List of Tables

Chapter One
Introduction

Recent changes in federal Medicaid laws have made it possible for states to offer Medicaid eligibility to a larger population at a lower cost to the state than was previously possible. Texas state officials have, with help of citizens, begun the search for funding alternatives which will make this expansion possible without requiring significant new state general revenue appropriations.

Three approaches are of particular interest. The first is the reallocation of dollars from existing state programs whose clientele could be served under Medicaid if eligibility were expanded. A system of voluntary contributions from hospitals to the state Medicaid budget is another option currently available. Finally, Texas can consider instituting a system of local funding for the program (or portions of the program) as a long-term alternative.

The exclusion of the medically indigent from federally funded medical assistance programs results in the costs of their care being shifted to state and local jurisdictions and to all paying patients through inflation of the prices they pay in compensation for the burden of non-paying patients. Expansion of Medicaid to a greater number of Texans will make it possible for a greater share of the burden of health care for the poor to be paid for with the federal tax dollars, instead of the state and local governments carrying the whole load.

The Case for Medicaid Expansion

Texas has historically limited its Medicaid

eligibility very strictly, in large part as a cost-saving measure. Prior to the changes introduced by the 1986 Omnibus Budget Reconciliation Act (OBRA 1986), the only way to get more Texans on Medicaid was to offer more Texans AFDC, entailing an increase in state spending on both the AFDC and Medicaid programs. OBRA 1986 created a window of opportunity for states to expand their coverage without having this expansion tied to AFDC levels (except via maintenance of effort requirements).

Other pressures have sharpened interest in Medicaid expansion. A survey of Texas hospitals found that they provided over $1.4 billion in uncompensated care in 1986.[1] There is a growing consensus, supported by a considerable body of evidence, that the bill for "uncompensated" care ultimately does end up being paid by the taxpayer. This may occur directly through taxes paid to support city, county and hospital district facilities, or indirectly through "cost-shifting", the inflation of health care prices to paying patients in public and private hospitals alike. The question apparently is not whether but how the taxpayers of Texas will pick up the tab for health care for the poor.

The increasingly active role of our state government in the provision of health care to the poor, notably in conjunction with the Indigent Health Care package of 1985, has resulted in a greatly heightened awareness not only of the magnitude of the uncompensated care burden on health care providers, but also of the broad dimensions of the population with unmet health care needs. This new level of commitment and spending, coinciding as it does with some of the strongest pressure ever to constrain state spending, has been the catalyst for a search for approaches to improving health care delivery which will minimize the need for additional state spending.

It is thought that a significant number of the people receiving uncompensated care in Texas are people who could qualify for Medicaid coverage if the state were to broaden its eligibility standards. Therefore, this argument continues, the state should do whatever is within its power to broaden those standards and thus capture federal matching dollars for Texas dollars which are "already being spent."

There also exists a growing sentiment that Texas should attempt to recapture a greater share of the dollars it sends off to Washington in the form of federal taxes. In 1985, Texans paid $1.59 in federal taxes for every $1.00 in federal grants-in-aid received by the state.[2] That same year, Texas, with 6.9% of the nation's population, received only 3.7% of all federal Medicaid expenditures. In contrast, New Yorkers, who make up 7.4% of the population, received 17.6% of the Medicaid budget,[3] and paid only $0.75 for every dollar in federal grants-in-aid which returned to the state. Californians paid $1.15 for every federal grants-in-aid dollar, and received 10% of federal Medicaid expenditures. The state and local share of matching costs for these federal programs increased by 50% from 1980 to 1985, while the actual federal grant disbursements increased by only 12%.[4] Figures for the ten most populous states are provided in Table 1.1.

A major cause of the imbalance between tax burden and federal benefits received has been Texas' choice to limit its participation in federally matched human service programs such as Medicaid. Even so, Medicaid is Texas' largest source of federal funding which is actually administered by the state (Medicare

Table 1.1
State's Population Compared to Federal Grants-in-Aid and Medicaid Expenditures Ten Most Populous States (1985)

State	% of U.S.[5] Population	% of 1985 Fed Medicaid Spending[6]	Fed Tax Burden per $ of Aid[7]
California	11.0%	10.0%	$1.15
New York	7.4	17.6	$0.75
Texas	6.9	3.7	$1.59
Pennsylvania	5.0	5.0	$0.97
Illinois	4.8	4.0	$1.15
Florida	4.8	2.6	$1.49
Ohio	4.5	4.5	$1.04
Michigan	3.8	4.0	$0.93
New Jersey	3.2	2.7	$1.42
North Carolina	2.6	2.1	$1.00

Sources: Texas Department of Human Services; Tax Foundation (as noted).

---

funding exceeds that of Medicaid),[8] and brought in over $1.1 million in 1987.[9] Our choice to limit spending at the state level for Medicaid has resulted in our not getting a proportionate share of the federal Medicaid pie and, in the process, has merely shifted the financial liability for indigent health care to other jurisdictions (including programs funded in part or in whole by the state) which are not eligible for matching federal funds.

The Texas legislature has demonstrated its desire to work towards a more efficient use of public funds via Medicaid expansion. The 70th legislature passed H.B. 1847, which amended the Maternal and Infant Health Improvement Act (MIHIA) of 1985, directing the Texas Department of Health to structure the MIHIA program in a manner which would maximize the generation of federal funds without a loss of service to the original target population. In addition, Lieutenant Governor Bill Hobby created a interim Select Committee on Medicaid and Family Services to study the options for expansion of Texas' Medicaid program. The committee held its first meeting in December of 1987.

The objective of this report is to describe the major funding issues which are embedded in the general question of Medicaid expansion. First, a description of the current program existing in Texas and of the parameters for expansion allowed under federal law is provided. This is followed by an discussion in Chapters Three and Four of some of the major state programs which are currently serving significant numbers of potentially Medicaid-eligible clients. The problems inherent in switching to a Medicaid-based system are explained, along with possible solutions to these problems.

The practical and political complexity of implementing a major expansion of Medicaid in Texas derives to a great extent from the fact that there are such a large number of interested groups (and, by extension, such a large amount of money) involved in the program. Policy makers have to deal not only with several large state agencies with overlapping interests and jurisdictions, but also with agents of a number of different major segments of the health care industry. Although all of the players have endorsed the general concept of Medicaid expansion, consensus on how that goal should be reached will require an understanding of the impact which expansion may have on all involved parties. Consensus building is not the only motive for recognizing the interests of health care providers. To the extent that inadequacies of reimbursement discourage participation in the Medicaid program, careful attention to provider payment programs may prove essential to insuring quality of and access to care for Medicaid recipients. Because the role of the health care providers is so critical, issues of concern to major industry groups are described in four short sections covering the reimbursement programs for hospitals, nursing homes, physicians and pharmacies.

In closing, the report takes a look at mechanisms for supplementing state general revenue funding of Medicaid with local funds. The final chapter provides indicators of the levels of expenditures by local and state jurisdictions on the provision of health care to Texans who cannot pay for it themselves, along with conclusions and recommendations for the future direction of the state's Medicaid program.

Notes

1. Texas Department of Health, Indigent Health Care Programs, Annual Report, 1988.(Pre-publication draft.)

2. Tax Foundation, "Federal Grants No Bargain in FY85 for 20 States Whose Average Tax `Cost' Per Aid Dollar Was $1.19," Washington, D.C., May 1986.(News Release.)

3. Texas Department of Human Services, "States' Population Compared to Federal Medicaid Expenditures," June, 1986. (Background information for presentation by Director of indigent health care program.)

4. Tax Foundation, "Federal Grants No Bargain in FY85 for 20 States Whose Average Tax `Cost' Per Aid Dollar Was $1.19," Washington, D.C., May 1986.(News Release.)

5. "Estimates of U.S. Resident Population by State: 1980, 1984 and 1985," The Number News, February 1986, reproduced by Texas Department of Human Services.

6. "Medicaid Assistance Payments - Federal Share, FFY 1985," Medicaid Financial Management Report, 1986, reproduced by Texas Department of Human Services.

7. Tax Foundation, "Federal Grants No Bargain in FY85 for 20 States Whose Average Tax `Cost' Per Aid Dollar Was $1.19," Washington, D.C., May 1986.(News Release.)

8. U.S. Congress, Select Committee on Aging, Medicare and Medicaid Reform: Protecting the Aged and Indigent in Texas, 99th Cong., 1st sess., 1985, p. 44.

9. Texas Department of Human Services, Fiscal Year 1987: Year-end Budget Report, Austin (December 17, 1987), p.3.

Chapter Two
Fundamentals of Medicaid

Medicaid is the name given to Title 19 of the Social Security Amendments of 1965. The Medicaid program is administered by the Health Care Financing Administration (HCFA) of the Department of Health and Human Services. Medicaid does not reimburse people for their medical expenses, but rather pays health care providers directly for services rendered to Medicaid-eligible persons. States are not required to offer Medicaid at all, but Arizona is the only state which does not offer the program. Since 1982, Arizona has offered a federally supplemented indigent health care program very similar to Medicaid. States which do offer Medicaid are required to provide it to certain groups of people as specified by federal code, and they are required to provide specific types of medical services. States also have the option of extending Medicaid coverage to certain other groups of people, and to offer certain other benefits or services under the program.

Medicaid Eligibility Standards

Mandatory Coverage

All state Medicaid programs are required to offer coverage to all persons who are receiving AFDC (Aid to Families with Dependent Children) or SSI (Supplemental Security Income). Title XIX also identifies a number of smaller groups for special eligibility standards, such as institutionalized persons (does not include inmates of correctional facilities), pregnant women who would be eligible for

AFDC if their child were already born, and others.[1] An explanation follows of how the two largest eligible groups, AFDC and SSI, are defined.

Table 2.1
Eligibility Categories Under
Texas Medicaid: 1988

AFDC-Related Categories	SSI Related Categories
* AFDC (Aid for Families with Dependent Children) Recipients - single parents and their dependent children (no adults from two-parent households unless one spouse is certified disabled).	**Supplemental Security Income (SSI) Recipients- individuals who are blind, disabled or over age 65 and whose income is less than the maximum SSI federal benefit rate of $340 per month (1987 level).
* Children up to age 19 from two-parent households whose family income and assets meet AFDC guidelines.	**Persons residing in Medicaid-approved nursing homes whose income is less than $658.65 per month (1987 level).
* Pregnant women whose income and assets meet AFDC guidelines (otherwise no single adults unless blind, disabled or over age 65).	
* Persons who fit any of the above three categories and whose income is too high to qualify for AFDC but is still less than 133% of the state's maximum AFDC grant. This is called the "Medically Needy" program.	

Source: Texas Department of Human Services, "Medicaid Eligibility in Texas," Austin, January 1988.(Summary data prepared for Congressman J.J. Pickle.)

The SSI program provides cash assistance to low income persons who are over 65, blind or disabled. The income standard for people in these categories is set by the federal government for the country as a whole. For example, in 1986 a blind, disabled or over-age-65 individual with an income of less than $336 monthly (about 79% of the federal poverty level) was eligible for SSI.[2] States can relax eligibility standards for SSI by supplementing the federal stipends with state money, but they cannot make the income standard more restrictive. In contrast, each state sets its own AFDC income standard (which cannot exceed the federal poverty level).

A characteristic of Medicaid which sets it apart from state and local social programs is that it is an entitlement program. Once the state has set eligibility standards, it has to take all comers who meet those standards. This means that the simplest approach a state can take to contain the cost of its Medicaid program is to limit services to some degree and, because SSI income eligibility levels are not very flexible, to set conservative (low) income standards for AFDC.

Texas currently sets this income standard at approximately 25% of the federal poverty level. Under this standard a mother with two dependent children whose adjusted income is even a dollar more than $184 a month is ineligible to receive AFDC.[3] This is obviously a much more conservative standard than that of SSI, so it is not surprising that Texas' Medicaid population is composed of a greater proportion of the elderly, blind and disabled than is true of the nation as a whole.[4] Also, although the number of Texans over age 65 is, at 9.4%, below the national average of 12.0%,[5] it has also been estimated that 43% of elderly Texans live below the Federal Poverty Level,[6] which may help account for the relatively high proportion of the Medicaid population which they comprise. This is a significant fact because the aged, blind and disabled population is a more "expensive" group: while in 1985 they accounted for less than 43% of Texans enrolled in Medicaid, they were responsible for over 80% of payments to health care providers.[7]

The Deficit Reduction Act of 1984 (DEFRA, P.L. 98-369) mandated Medicaid coverage of pregnant women, married or single, who meet AFDC income and asset guidelines but who do not have an AFDC eligible child in their household. The law also required states to cover children up to age 5 who live in households whose income meets AFDC guidelines but who do not meet the AFDC definition of deprived children because there are two parents present in the home, and extended coverage automatically to infants born of mothers who are eligible for and currently receiving Medicaid. Texas implemented these provisions in October of 1984 under the program called CPW (for Children and Pregnant Women). This program exceeds the coverage changes which were mandated by DEFRA by also adding optional coverage of children from age six to age 19 living in two-parent families which meet the AFDC income and asset guidelines.[8]

Optional Coverage

Title XIX also identifies a number of other groups to which states may offer Medicaid coverage if they choose. A number of these categories are designed to allow states to assure that people who are receiving benefits from certain social programs do not lose their Medicaid eligibility in the process. For example, a mother who is eligible for AFDC (and thus for Medicaid) while she is paying for and deducting the costs of child care from her income is protected from losing her Medicaid benefits should she begin to receive public child care assistance which leaves her income just high enough to keep her off the AFDC rolls.[9] There are also provisions which protect coverage of those enrolled in Medicaid-qualified Health Maintenance Organizations and recipients of home and community based Medicaid services which exist in restricted areas by special arrangement with HCFA.[10]

There are several other major categories of persons to whom states can offer Medicaid. States are allowed to grant Medicaid coverage to all persons who would be eligible to receive AFDC if the state were exercising all of the options available under federal AFDC guidelines. This includes children only up to age 21 from two-parent families (of any employment status) who would be eligible for AFDC/Medicaid on the basis of family income alone (states are not required to offer AFDC to such families) and entire two-parent families in which the principal earner is unemployed.[11] The coverage of children between age six and age 19 under the CPW program which was described above is possible because of this option. There are also eligibility options for institutionalized persons who would otherwise be receiving Medicaid.[12]

Medically Needy Programs

Further options are available to state Medicaid programs under the "medically needy" categories (all of the above-mentioned eligibility categories are commonly referred to as the "categorically needy"). Basically the medically needy options allow extension of Medicaid coverage to persons who would qualify for AFDC or SSI except that their income is slightly higher than state standards. The maximum income level a state can set for Medically Needy eligibility is 133 1/3% of the states maximum AFDC income level (which cannot exceed Federal poverty levels).

Texas implemented its first medically needy (MN) program in January of 1985. Covered at present are pregnant women (married or single), children from two-parent families who do not qualify as deprived children under AFDC (just as explained above under the CPW program), children who do qualify as deprived children under AFDC, and the caretakers of deprived children. Since the federal income limit for eligibility under a MN program is 133 1/3% of a state's maximum AFDC grant, the upper income limit for Texas' MN program is 34% of the federal poverty level.[13] To illustrate, in 1987 a single mother with two dependent children who earned no more than $184 per month (and met AFDC asset limits) would have received both AFDC and Medicaid. If her income fell between $184 and $267 per month (again, assets must meet AFDC guidelines) she would qualify for Medicaid under the medically Needy program, but would receive no cash assistance.[14]

There is also, however, a mechanism referred to as "spend down" which allows a family whose income exceeds this level to qualify for Medicaid coverage if family medical expenses exceed the difference between household income and the MN income threshold for six consecutive months.[15]

New Options: OBRA 1986

The effect of these income level restrictions in the past has been to make it impossible for most states to expand their Medicaid covered population without also expanding their AFDC programs. However, in 1986 the 99th U.S. Congress passed legislation as part of the Omnibus Budget Reconciliation Act (OBRA: P.L. 99-509) which grants the states new latitude in extending Medicaid coverage to AFDC and SSI ineligible residents. The essence of this legislation was to allow states to offer Medicaid coverage to certain categories of persons with incomes all the way up to the federal poverty level regardless of what the states' maximum AFDC income levels are. An important stipulation of the law is that states which take advantage of the new options must maintain AFDC payments at or above the levels which were in effect on April 17, 1986.[16]

The first category includes pregnant women and infants up to age one, and (to be phased in one year at a time) children up to age five who are under 100% of federal poverty level.[17] States must exercise this option before they may offer coverage to any of the other categories created under the new law. States which do so may then offer Medicaid coverage to elderly and disabled residents up to 100% of federal poverty level, or as an alternative, they may instead choose to pay the Medicare cost-sharing obligations of their elderly and disabled Medicare recipients up to 100% of federal poverty level.[18]

Several other noteworthy changes came out of OBRA. Eligibility status of aliens has been clarified. Emergency medical services provided to illegal aliens who in every respect other than their citizenship status would qualify for Medicaid will henceforth be eligible for federal matching funds. Emergency services are defined to specifically include labor and delivery services.[19] Furthermore, the Immigration Reform and Control Act of 1986 provides that all aliens who qualify for legalization under the act will be eligible to apply for Medicaid five years from the time they are granted legal status. Certain categories of these legal aliens will be exempt from the five-year waiting period, namely: aged, blind and disabled persons, children under age 18, pregnant women for their pregnancy-related needs only, and Cuban or Haitian applicants. Emergency medical services will also be covered without a waiting period.[20]

Also new under OBRA is the option for states to offer Medicaid services to pregnant women during a period of "presumptive eligibility"; that is, as soon as a health care provider who is Medicaid approved has made a preliminary judgement based on income information that the woman is eligible for Medicaid, but before the state agency administering Medicaid has made a decision regarding that woman's application. The women must make official application for Medicaid coverage within 14 days of these services in order for presumed eligibility to continue.[21] Since states have up to 45 days to render decisions on Medicaid applications, this provision helps eliminate delays in obtaining prenatal care. Also of great importance is the stipulation that services rendered during the presumptive eligibility period to women who are ultimately found to be ineligible will still be paid for by Medicaid.

Table 2.2
Comparison of Asset Requirements

	AFDC Program	Food Stamps	SSI Program
Resource Limit	$1,000 per Family	$2,000 per Family	$1,900 per person; $2,850 per couple.
Homestead	Usual Texas residence exempted:rural < 200 acres; urban < 1 acre	Usual Residence exempted	Exempted if individual, spouse, or dependent lives in residence.
Other Real Property	Current Equity Value is counted.	Current Equity Value is counted.	Current Equity Value is counted.
Life Insurance	Cash value is counted.	Cash value of life ins. and pension funds exempted.	Face value exempt only if < $1500
Vehicle	Value of one vehicle exempt if EQUITY < $1500; if greater, only excess is counted. Equity of other vehicles is counted.	Exempt primary vehicle if market value < $4500 (count excess). Greater of mkt. value over $4500 or equity for other vehicles.	Exempt one vehicle if current retail value < or =$4500. Excess is counted.
Liquid Assets	Counted.	Counted.	Counted.

Source: Texas Department of Human Services, "Comparison of Resource Requirements," Austin, February 1988. (Materials prepared for Select Committee on Medicaid and Family Services.)

OBRA 1986 also authorizes states to completely dispose of the use of an assets test for eligibility determinations of pregnant women and children under age five. The law further stipulates that if a state does use an asset test for pregnant women, it may not use a standard more restrictive than the one used by SSI. Since the SSI assets test is more liberal than that used in Texas' AFDC program, this provision alone would make it easier for pregnant women to qualify for Medicaid.[22] A comparison of the assets requirements of the AFDC, Food Stamp and SSI Programs is provided in Table 2.2.

Proponents of adoption of the option to waive the test entirely point out that the assets test consumes a great deal of time and is complex and difficult to document. At present in Texas only about 2.44% of applicants for the Medicaid Pregnant Women's program are rejected due to excess assets.[23] In fact, it is more common for applicants to be rejected because they cannot document adequately their assets than because those assets actually exceed the standards.[24]

If a state does adopt a more generous asset standard for pregnant women, it may be applied to all pregnant women with incomes less than whatever maximum the state chooses. In this way, a woman who loses AFDC purely because of excess assets (but whose income still meets AFDC standards) may be able to retain her Medicaid eligibility if those assets do not exceed the special Pregnant Women's asset test.

Another significant option made available to states under the legislation is what is referred to as "continuous eligibility". If a state so chooses, it may allow any woman who is certified eligible for

Medicaid coverage at the onset of pregnancy to remain eligible until 60 days after the delivery of her child; that is, she will not be required to recertify her eligibility.[25] The goal of this option is to eliminate the interruption of prenatal care due to slight increases in income which, while sufficient to make the mother ineligible for Medicaid, are unlikely to make private insurance available to her.

Provisions under OBRA and the Omnibus Drug Act of 1986 clarified the Medicaid eligibility status of homeless individuals. According to OBRA, states may not impose any residency requirement that excludes from coverage any otherwise qualified individual who resides in the state, regardless of whether that person can provide a permanent or fixed address.[26] The Omnibus Drug Act further requires that states have in place a mechanism for making Medicaid cards available to the homeless by January 1, 1987.[27]

Further Options: OBRA 1987

The Omnibus Budget Reconciliation Act of 1987 (OBRA 1987), which was signed into law on December 22, 1987, contained provisions which further expanded eligibility options initiated in OBRA 1986. Effective July 1, 1988, states may extend Medicaid coverage of pregnant women and infants under one year of age to persons with incomes up to 185% of the federal poverty level. States are granted the option, with specific limitations, of imposing a premium or co-payment for services to the pregnant women and children in this group with incomes which exceed 150% of the federal poverty level after child care expenses have been deducted. States are also given the option to immediately offer coverage to the children up to age five under 100% of federal poverty level who were targeted by OBRA 1986, eliminating the phase-in period contained in that legislation.[28]

OBRA 1987 extended the mandatory coverage initiated by DEFRA of children whose family incomes and assets meet state AFDC guidelines, but who do not meet the AFDC definition of deprived children. The new law requires that states cover children up to age eight who fall into this category;[29] DEFRA mandated coverage through age six. As previously noted, Texas covers such children through age 19 under the CPW program, so this change in the law will have no impact here.

OBRA 1987 included a provision that extends the Medicaid coverage of pregnant women to the end of the calendar month in which a 60-day period beginning with her delivery date falls. State are prohibited from stipulating that women and children who enroll in Medicaid under these optional coverage provisions to also be required to apply for AFDC as a condition of receiving Medicaid. A maintenance of effort clause prohibits states which implement the optional coverage from lowering their AFDC standard from that level which was in effect on July 1, 1987.[30]

Services Covered Under Medicaid

Required services

All states are required to cover certain services under Medicaid, although they are allowed to place some limits on the extent of these services. Required services include in- and out-patient hospital, rural health clinic, lab and X-ray, skilled nursing facility, home health care, family planning, physician care, medical transportation, nurse-midwife care, and early and periodic screening, diagnosis and treatment of physical and mental defects in eligible persons under age 21 (referred to as EPSDT).[31]

Table 2.3
Status of Medicaid Services
In Texas: 1988

ALL Medicaid programs must pay for certain services to Medicaid recipients, including:	**Optional services Texas Medicaid will NOT pay for include:**
-inpatient and outpatient hospital bills -lab and X-ray bills -skilled nursing facilities -home health care programs -family planning programs -doctors' bills -a program of regular check-ups for minors	-physical, occupational, or speech therapy -routine dental care -dentures -private duty nursing -clinic services -inpatient psychiatric care for those under 22 or over 65 -other diagnostic, screening, preventive and rehabilitative services
Other services may be covered at a state's option. Optional services offered in Texas include:	
-prescriptions (three per month in Texas) -optometry and eyeglasses -emergency medical services -medically needed oral surgery -podiatry -hearing aids and prosthetic devices -day surgery -intermediate care (many nursing homes) -limited rehabilitation services	

Source: Texas Department of Human Services, State Plan Under Title XIX of the Social Security Act, sec. 2,3.

Optional Services

A number of other services may be provided at state option. As with the mandatory services, states may limit the extent of provision. Texas provides prescription drugs (limited to 3 per month), optometry and eyeglasses, emergency medical services, chiropractic care, prostheses, hearing aids, oral surgery for broken jaws and life-threatening infection only, podiatry, limited rehabilitative services, intermediate care, and ambulatory surgery (outpatient surgery).[32]

Texas does not cover physical, occupational or speech therapy, private duty nursing, clinic services, routine dental care, dentures, or inpatient psychiatric services for those under 22 or over 65 (these are the only two groups which could be eligible for inpatient psychiatric services under federal Medicaid guidelines). Also uncovered in Texas is a range of services which may be covered under the umbrella of "other diagnostic, screening, preventive and rehabilitation services."[33] Adoption of several of these uncovered optional services is being examined currently, both as a possible tool for implementation of eligibility expansion in the area of maternal and child health and also as a way to inject new federal dollars into the mental health and mental retardation programs.

Program Design Requirements

There are several provisions of the Social Security Act which aim to ensure that states do not discriminate either among qualified providers of medical services or among those eligible for services. Section 1902 of Title XIX requires that each state's

Medicaid program must make comparable services available to all categorically needy recipients. Medically needy recipients' services may be less extensive but cannot be more extensive. States are also required to make all Medicaid services available on a statewide basis; that is, every type of Medicaid service which a state provides must be available to all eligible residents, and may not be restricted to residents of certain localities. A third provision is that recipients be given freedom to utilize any qualified medical provider they choose except in a few very limited circumstances. To illustrate, under most normal circumstances a state cannot require Medicaid recipients to utilize particular public clinics or public hospitals. These three requirements are commonly referred to as "comparability", "statewideness", and "freedom of choice".

These requirements pose problems for specialized medical assistance programs such as health maintenance organizations (HMOs) or "channeling" programs (like Texas' MIHIA program) which target high-risk pregnant women. HMOs tend to operate on a local or regional basis, which would violate the statewideness requirement of Title XIX. Any program which targets a population for services based on a special medical need is at risk of violating the comparability requirement if it offers a level of services to its clients which is more extensive than that offered to other Medicaid eligibles on any basis other than medical need. Either type of program would normally be in violation of freedom of choice requirements if recipients were limited, for example, to certain HMO facilities or high-risk specialists.

<u>Waivers of Design Requirements</u>

In recognition of the cost-saving potential represented by programs such as those mentioned above, amendments to Medicaid have been made in recent years which, subject to HCFA approval, allow states to waive requirements of freedom of choice, comparability, and statewideness.[34] OBRA 1981 authorized the granting of freedom of choice waivers to allow states to require Medicaid recipients to utilize specified providers (emergency services are excluded) deemed efficient and cost effective.[35] Califorinia and Illinois have used such waivers extensively for inpatient hospitalization. Providers submit bids on a area-by-area basis, and enough of the low bidders are granted contracts to guarantee access to service by all area recipients. OBRA 1986 specifically allows states to establish waiver programs which target groups which are at high risk of requiring hospitalization, and specifically mentions persons with AIDS or AIDS related complex as an example of such a high-risk group.[36] Waivers must be demonstrable as being "cost-effective, efficient, and consistent with the objectives of the Medicaid program."[37]

An important adaptation of Medicaid design requirements was created by the Consolidated Omnibus Budget Reconciliation Act of 1985 (COBRA: P.L. 99-272). The law stipulates that "a state may provide, as medical assistance, case management services under the plan without regard to the requirements of section 1902(a)(1) [statewideness] and section 1902(a)(10)(B) [comparability] [and] shall not restrict the choice of the individual to receive medical assistance in violation of section 1902(a)(23) [freedom of choice]."

This provision has been interpreted as treating case management systems as an optional service (like clinic services or dentures) which states may choose to offer. A state must submit a State Plan Amendment to HCFA for approval to add an optional service. The addition of optional services via State Plan Amendment is generally considered to be much quicker and less arduous than the waiver approach.

Design requirements, waiver options and the potential uses of optional services are important elements which define both the current structure of state Medicaid plans and the potential for adjustments to those plans. The practical and political feasibility of many Medicaid expansion programs depends heavily on a state's ability to find artful ways to achieve local program goals while remaining within the limits required by the federal program. The uses of these approaches by other states and the prospects for taking advantage of those approaches in Texas are discussed in Chapters Three and Four.

Notes

1. 42 CFR Sec. 435.110-435.136.

2. U.S. House of Reps., Committee on Ways and Means, Background Material and Data on Programs Within the Jurisdiction of the Committee on Ways and Means, 1986 ed.,99th Congress 2d sess., March 3, 1986, p. 468.

3. State Medicaid Information Center of National Governors' Association; "Annualized Medicaid Eligibility Thresholds- AFDC, Medically Needy, SSI- As Percent of Poverty," December 1986. (Chart.)

4. M. Gornick et.al.,"Twenty Years of Medicare and Medicaid: Covered Populations, Use of benefits, and Program expenditures," Health Care Financing Review, 1985 annual supplement, p. 15.

5. U.S. Bureau of the Census, "Resident Population by Age and State: 1985," Statistical Abstract of the United States: 1987, 107th edition, Washington, D.C., 1986, p. 23.

6. U.S. Congress, House Committee on Ways and Means, Background Material and Data on Programs Within the Jurisdiction of the Committee on Ways and Means, 99th Cong., 2nd sess., March 3, 1986, p. 468.

7. Congressional Budget Office, "Medicaid Medical Vendor Payments by Maintenance Assistance Status of Recipient, Fiscal Year 1985," May 1, 1986. (Computer printout.)

8. Texas Department of Human Services, "AFDC-Related Medicaid Programs," January 1986. (Memorandum prepared for U.S. Congressman J.J. Pickle.)

9. 42 CFR Sec. 435.220.

10. 42 CFR Sec. 435.212, 435.217.

11. 42 CFR Sec. 435.223.

12. 42 CFR Sec 435.211, 435.231.

13. Ibid.

14. Texas Department of Human Services, "AFDC-Related Medicaid Programs," January 1986. (Memorandum prepared for U.S. Congressman J.J. Pickle.)

15. Texas Department of Human Services, "AFDC-Related Medicaid Programs," January 1986. (Memorandum prepared for U.S. Congressman J.J. Pickle.)

16. Sixth Omnibus Budget Reconciliation Act of 1986, P.L.99-509, Sec. 9401.

17. Ibid.

18. Ibid., Sec. 9402-9403.

19. Ibid., Sec. 9406.

20. Immigration Reform and Control Act of 1986, P.L. 99-603.

21. P.L. 99-509, Sec. 9407.

22. P.L. 99-507, section 9401.

23. Texas Department of Health and Texas Department of Human Services, "Maternal and Infant Health Care for Low-Income Texans: Memorandum of Understanding," Austin (March 1988), p. I-9.(Final Report to Commissioners.)

24. Sara Rosenbaum, "Medicaid Eligibility for Pregnant Women: Reforms Contained in the Sixth Omnibus Budget Reconciliation Act," (Children's Defense Fund, Washington, D.C., April 1987) pp. 8-9, 23.

25. P.L. 99-507, section 9501.

26. Ibid., Sec. 9405.

27. Omnibus Drug Act of 1986, P.L. 99-570, Sec. 10005 (b).

28. The Omnibus Budget Reconciliation Act of 1987, P.L. 100-203, Section 4101.

29. Ibid.

30. Ibid.

31. Texas Department of Human Services, State Plan Under Title XIX of the Social Security Act Medical Assistance Program, attachment 3.1A and attachment to same.

32. Ibid.

33. Ibid.

34. 42 CFR, sec. 431.54, 431.55; Social Security Act, Title XIX, sec. 1915; 42 USC, sec. 1396n.

35. The Omnibus Budget Reconciliation Act of 1981, P.L.99-35, sec. 2175.

36. P.L. 99-509, sec.9411.

37. 42 CFR, sec. 431.55(a).

Chapter Three
Targeted for Change:
The MIHIA Program

Barriers to Expansion

One goal of Medicaid expansion plans for Texas is to realize the potential which expansion holds for replacing state and local funding of health care services with federal funding. Accomplishing this goal will not be administratively simple in any case, but certain state programs have been identified which are promising targets for expansion. Programs which are the most likely candidates are those which serve groups of people who could be covered by Medicaid under options available to the state. The challenge to Texas is to devise approaches to expansion which will assure not only that Medicaid coverage will provide the same quality of care as the state programs, but also that the switch to broader Medicaid coverage can be accomplished in such a way that new federal revenues will completely offset or even exceed any new state and local spending.

Medicaid design requirements limit the extent to which a state can control either what services a recipient gets or where he gets them. One of the biggest concerns when the state considers applying money from a state funded program to the Medicaid budget is that in theory there is no guarantee that Medicaid recipients will keep using the same health care providers that they did under the state program. This in turn means that some amount of the new federal matching money could conceivably end up in the hands of private health care providers. If a large enough number of Medicaid patients were to shift to private providers, expansion of Medicaid would not be budget neutral for Texas government even though it was bringing in more dollars to the state in absolute terms (unless, of course, the cost of services were to drop significantly).

The same Medicaid design requirements may also make it difficult to ensure that targeted groups of patients such as high risk groups receive the same intensity of services under Medicaid as they did under state programs which are not bound by those freedom of choice constraints.

Other states have run up against these built-in limitations of the Medicaid program, and solutions are being found. One of the most powerful tools available to the states is the latitude which they are given in creating state-specific qualifications for being a Medicaid provider. These standards may include the numbers and qualifications of staff, the scope of available services and facilities, and financial reporting requirements for providers. Carefully tailored provider requirements may make it possible for Texas to reallocate resources to the Medicaid program with a minimum amount of financial risk. Some of the state programs which are under consideration for coordination with Medicaid are described in this chapter and the next.

The MIHIA Program

The Maternal and Infant Health Improvement Act (MIHIA) was passed by the 69th Texas Legislature, and resulted in the creation of a program administered by the Texas Department of Health (TDH) which has improved the quality of maternity services to the poor in two ways. First, the program provides basic prenatal care to women up to 200% of federal poverty level. The second component of the program provides comprehensive prenatal care to women under 100% of poverty who are determined to have high risk pregnancies. Care and follow-up for the infants up to one year of age of these high-risk mothers is also provided. The program is administered through contracts with local providers (there were 32 such contracts in 1987[1]) who delivered approximately 10,000 babies under the program in 1987.[2] TDHS estimates that there will be approximately 36,640 births to women under 100% of poverty in Texas in 1989, and they anticipate that 11,000 would be served by MIHIA if it continued in its present status.[3] Based on these figures, MIHIA would be anticipated to serve approximately 30% of the eligible population. However, this does not mean that only 30% of that population is served, since additional births are funded under the Title V Maternal and Child Health Block Grant. MIHIA contracts are located in many of the most populous areas of the state. The Panhandle, far East Texas and far West Texas have noticeably scanty MIHIA coverage, though the programs in Midland and Taylor counties in West Texas respectively cover 17 and 18 county areas.[4]

The 70th Texas legislature with H.B. 1847 amended MIHIA by directing the Health Department to structure the program in a manner which would maximize the amount of federal matching funds generated without a loss of service to the original target population.[5] This legislation came about as a response to the 1986 OBRA option allowing coverage of pregnant women up to 100% of poverty. Because TDHS is the agency which actually administers Medicaid, the two agencies (TDHS and TDH) must work together to come up with a plan which will meet the requirements of the state law. An interagency steering committee adopted a memorandum of understanding (MOU) effective January 1, 1988 regarding the potential coordination of MIHIA and Medicaid.

The most serious problem to be dealt with in "Medicaidizing" the MIHIA program is finding a way to insure that pregnant women continue to receive a quality of care once they become Medicaid recipients equal to what they would have under the state's program. Because the care of newborns and infants with health problems is some of the most expensive in all of medicine, the provision of good prenatal care to low-income mothers can save Texans a good deal of money.

Studies comparing the pregnancies of women under Medicaid with those of women in special prenatal care case management programs have reported significantly poorer pregnancy outcomes for the Medicaid mothers. In a North Carolina study of births in one county in 1984, the low birth weight rate for women in the health department's perinatal program was 8.3%, compared to 19.3% for the Medicaid mothers.[6] A study of Medi-Cal recipients reported a 4.7% low birthweight rate for women enrolled in a case management program, and a 7% rate for the control group Medi-Cal mothers.[7] Both these and other studies conclude that the reason for the poorer outcome for Medicaid babies is not substandard care by Medicaid physicians. Medicaid, except when specifically engineered to do otherwise, simply lacks any mechanism to guarantee that recipients will get needed services on a timely basis. In fact, it is the greatly improved access to ancillary services such as education, home visits, nutritional assessment and counseling, and referral to appropriate social services which is thought to be responsible for the improved outcome under case management, and not any difference in the number or quality of prenatal physician visits.[8]

Two Approaches to "Medicaidizing" MCH Programs: Case Management With and Without a Waiver

In light of evidence such as the studies mentioned above, much of the movement towards implementation of H.B. 1847 has focused on the search for a mechanism to preserve within the context of the Medicaid program the case managed prenatal care system which MIHIA has begun building. Some of the regulatory and administrative hurdles which must be cleared in order to effect such a program are explained below, along with some alternative approaches to clearing those hurdles.

Waiver Programs

In August of 1986 HCFA and the U.S. Public Health Service issued a joint memorandum which indicated their endorsement of the use of waiver services for programs which target special populations. The stated purpose of the memorandum was "to assist the state Maternal and Child Health agency and the state Medicaid agency in developing collaborative relationships which address certain innovations possible in the state Medicaid plan."[9] The issuance details the waiver process and cites the South Carolina High Risk Channeling Program as a model of how waivers can be used to allow Medicaid recipients to utilize a high risk channeling program. Concluding remarks note that "virtually any possible model of case managed health care" could be applied to a high risk program, "provided the program meets the regulatory requirements for cost effectiveness, access to services, quality of care, and program impact in 42 CFR 431.55(b)."[10]

All state Medicaid agencies do not share the enthusiasm for waiver programs which HCFA communicated in the above-mentioned memorandum. A common perception of those involved in waiver programs at the state level is that HCFA's requirements for documentation, particularly of cost-effectiveness, are overly rigorous and difficult to satisfy. States are required to identify both the sources and the magnitudes of potential savings offered by a program, which can be difficult when a program exists only on paper. HCFA has also been known to object to the use of savings estimates which are based on projections of need for the proposed services. They reason that if a waiver program serves more people than did the system which it replaces, the program may end up costing HCFA more overall even if the per-client cost is reduced. Although this "cold-bed" approach clearly may save money in the short run, it has a punitive effect on states which may wish to use the waiver approach to upgrade previously inadequate services.

Although HCFA must either approve a waiver proposal or respond with a request for further information within 90 days, it is not uncommon for the waiver approval process to take more than one year, and in some cases even longer. For example, the South

Carolina waiver program touted by HCFA was requested on November 1, 1984. Final approval was granted October 18, 1985, to be effective 90 days from that date.[11] The time a state waits for approval is in addition to whatever time was previously required to develop necessary political consensus and/or enabling legislation compounded by the time required to develop the waiver proposal itself for submission. To avoid this delay, states may look for alternatives to waivers whenever feasible.

The waiver program is one tool which Texas may need to utilize in its search for strategies to maximize federal match for existing appropriations. The waiver approach has in its favor the power to allow a program to restrict clients to desired services and providers to the greatest degree possible under Title XIX. Use of an approved waiver system would also assure the state somewhat that HCFA would not disallow (refuse to match) expended funds for the program. On the down side, it would seem that this approach could delay unacceptably the actual implementation of a plan, or make it difficult to adapt the program should changes be indicated as time passed.

In April of 1986, the state of South Carolina implemented a perinatal channelling project for Medicaid recipients. Impetus for the project was provided to some extent by the successful experience which the state has had since 1976 with its High Risk Perinatal Program (HRPP) for medically indigent women (those with no source of third party payment for medical care). Though the OBRA 1986 options did not exist at the time the waiver program was conceived and thus were not a motivating factor in the program's creation, the state's decision to implement coverage of pregnant women and children up to 100% of poverty has broadened the scope of the program considerably.

The South Carolina High Risk Channeling Program (HRCP) restricts clients to providers with specialized skills or facilities and thus requires a freedom of choice waiver under section 1915(b) of Title XIX. For example, the HRCP restricts high risk pregnant women to using board certified OB-GYNs and Level II or III hospitals (higher level ratings indicate enhanced staff levels and technical resources). This system did encounter some resistance from General and Family practitioners, from Level I hospitals and from qualified OB-GYNs who because of their distance from Level II or III hospitals must send their high risk Medicaid clients elsewhere for delivery.[12] However, for the most part the creation of the High Risk Channeling Project was facilitated by the presence of broad based support from the Hospital Association, State Medical Association, pediatricians and perinatologists organizations, the Governor's office and South Carolina's Congressional delegation.[13] This unity of purpose may have been attributable to a desire to reduce South Carolina's infant mortality rate, which was the highest in the nation as recently as 1983.[14] The level of consensus behind a waiver program is likely to be critical to its success.

An evaluation of the HRCP's first year performed by the Department of Health Administration of the School of Public Health at the University of South Carolina has concluded that even at this early date, there are significant discernible cost savings which can be attributed to the project. The channeling of high-risk Medicaid mothers into higher level hospitals is naturally associated with increased costs for both mother and infant; however, the South Carolina study found that savings due to reduced transfers of infants to higher level hospitals came to about $10,000 per month, which more than offset the increased hospitalization costs of approximately $2,000 per month.[15] The HRCP data was sufficient to support the assignment of a specific figure due to savings from improved birth outcomes. Counties with low participation rates in the program had significantly poorer overall birth outcomes and significantly longer lengths of stay in expensive neonatal intensive care units, but the authors acknowledge that it is not possible to attribute these differences to the program.[16]

Case Management as an Optional Service

A slightly different approach to adaptation of a perinatal program to encompass Medicaid clients is being considered in a number of states. North Carolina has expanded eligibility up to the federal poverty level for pregnant women and children up to age two. The Maternal and Child Health division of the state Division of Health Services is working with the Division of Medical Assistance to promote a rigorous case management system which, in conjunction with the eligibility expansion, is expected to virtually replace the existing perinatal program.[17] The legal basis for this plan is the case management provision of COBRA which was described in Chapter Two.

Under the program, clients may choose any qualified case manager, or may forego the use of case management altogether without jeopardizing Medicaid coverage. Because participation is optional for the client, and because clients may choose between Medicaid qualified service providers, the program does not require a waiver. Under North Carolina guidelines, case managers or "Maternity Care Coordinators" (MCCS) must be either Registered Nurses or Social Workers, and they must be employed by some entity which has signed an agreement with the DHS and is a Medicaid provider.[18] As a result, in the early stages of implementation case management has been provided largely by local, rural or community health centers, mirroring the previously existing perinatal network. Since case managers are available in the same locations where many newly eligible Medicaid recipients have gone in the past, participation requires no extra effort by the client; in addition, a vigorous outreach program is included in the plan. Outreach is also aimed at making physicians aware of the program so that they can refer their Medicaid patients. Guidelines are broad enough, however, to include private physicians or group practices as case managers in the future if they should care to participate.[19]

North Carolina officials hope to avoid disharmony with the medical community by not restricting freedom of choice to the degree that their neighbors to the south have. They feel that their existing informal perinatal network is quite sound. Using the enhancement of case management coupled with the application of standards of risk assessment currently set by the American College of Obstetrics and Gynecology, they expect to attain high quality risk management without a waiver program.[20]

Implications for MIHIA

Actual implementation of H.B. 1847 is still in the early stages. The challenge facing the TDH-TDHS coordinators was to develop an approach which complies with Medicaid requirements and also protects the high-risk targeting capacity of MIHIA. If maximizing the influx of federal dollars were their only priority, the agencies could agree to apply MIHIA's funding to the state Medicaid pot, and add coverage of pregnant women and children up to some income level commensurate with the estimated increase in available funds. This would have the effect of providing third-party coverage for many more women and children, and would help ease the burden of uncompensated care on Texas hospitals. What would be lost is a formal mechanism to channel women to a level of perinatal care appropriate to their individual health needs. It seems unlikely that the state will retreat on a commitment to quality perinatal care so recently expressed in the form of the creation of MIHIA. In addition, the MIHIA program offers basic prenatal care to women up to 200% of federal poverty level, while Medicaid coverage can be expanded to 185% of poverty at best, so a segment of MIHIA's population would still be ineligible for Medicaid even under the most generous possible income standards.

Texas' Medicaid system will require some modification if some of the character of MIHIA is to be retained. The waiver option may not be a practical tactic in Texas. Documentation of the cost-effectiveness of a state-wide program will not be simple for such a large state. Also, the sensitivity of physicians and proprietary hospitals to any perceived threat of restrictions on freedom of choice should not be discounted. The 1915(b) waiver clearly states that freedom of choice may be limited only on the basis of intensity and quality of care, and may not discriminate on any grounds unrelated to demonstrated effectiveness and efficiency. For example, a state may limit high-risk Medicaid mothers to higher level hospitals, but may not explicitly limit them to public hospitals. Nevertheless, considerable apprehension among provider groups does exist, and an approach closer to that of North Carolina may be practically and politically easier to realize in Texas.

It may be possible for Texas to retain many of the desirable characteristics of MIHIA via the addition of optional services which we do not currently offer. If case management were offered as a service, entities which are currently MIHIA contractors could conceivably provide case management and bill Medicaid directly for their services. Since states are allowed to offer case management without being considered in violation of comparability requirements, there is reason to believe that the goals of MIHIA could be addressed by such a program.

In a similar vein, the Children's Defense Fund has for some time advocated the adoption of maternity, pediatric and primary health care clinic services, saying that as Medicaid providers the clinics could contract with off-premises physicians to provide services to the Medicaid eligible. The clinics would bill Medicaid and make payments to those physicians. This would eliminate the necessity for physicians to become direct Medicaid providers themselves.[21] While a majority of current MIHIA physician providers are also Medicaid providers,[22] it is possible that this flexibility will make participation in provision of care to these patients attractive to more doctors. Since problems of increased liability and difficulties in obtaining malpractice insurance create a disincentive for doctors to serve indigent high risk patients, this is an important consideration.

New provider requirements for case managers and/or for clinics can be written in such a way as to insure a level of expertise in keeping with MIHIA standards. Changes in some existing provider requirements may make it possible to channel higher risk patients to appropriate levels of care without violating freedom of choice. In all, the prospects for protecting the integrity of MIHIA via creative use of legitimate Medicaid options are favorable.

Recent Proposals for Implementation of H.B. 1847

TDH and TDHS in March of 1988 presented a report to the commissioners of the two agencies which included the memorandum of understanding required by the law.[23] This report included the recommendations of the work groups created by the interagency steering committee. On March 30, 1988 the Select Committee on Medicaid and Family Services proposed a set of draft recommendations, all having to do with the adoption of maternal and child eligibility expansion. For the most part, the recommendations of the Select Committee echoed the MIHIA proposals. Major recommendations of the MIHIA steering committee are described below. Areas in which the proposals of the Select Committee differed are noted.

1) OBRA-86 coverage of pregnant women and

children up to age one should be adopted up to a minimum of 100% of poverty.

Subject to availability of appropriations, coverage of older children could be added at the same income level.[24] The Select Committee recommended that coverage be granted immediately to children up to age three, with subsequent phase-in of children up to "school age".[25]

2) The resource (asset) standards used by the Food Stamp program should be adopted for this population of women.

The work group noted that the complete elimination of the resource standard would have a beneficial effect on continuity of care, would eliminate a possible source of error penalties for the state, and would simplify the application process and thereby eliminate a psychological barrier to participation. However, the work group felt that public opinion would run strongly against the elimination of an assets test, and opted to choose the less restrictive Food Stamp guidelines as a compromise measure.[26]

3) Continuous eligibility should be adopted for all pregnant Medicaid recipients.

The report noted that continuous eligibility might increase the willingness of providers to serve Medicaid clients, since they would no longer run a risk that the patient will lose coverage at some point during her pregnancy. The option would also absolve the state of responsibility for monitoring the income of pregnant recipients after initial qualification, and would thereby eliminate the risk of incurring income-based federal error penalties.[27]

4) Presumptive eligibility should receive further study before any implementation.

OBRA 1986 established specific guidelines for presumptive eligibility (PE) providers. To qualify as a PE provider, an entity must be (1) a qualified Medicaid provider _and_ (2) be either a hospital outpatient clinic or a freestanding clinic (this includes rural health clinics) _and_ (3) receive funding from or participate in one of the following: the federal Community Health Center program, the Migrant Health Center program, the Title V MCH Block Grant, the Special Supplemental Food Program for Women, Infants and Children (WIC), the Commodity Supplemental Food Program, or the state's perinatal health program, which in Texas is MIHIA.[28] Although a number of potentially eligible PE providers exist in Texas, many of them could only participate with the addition of clinic and rural health services to the Medicaid State Plan. The addition of those services in combination with the above mentioned federally imposed PE guidelines could have significant channelling effects. The analysis of PE by the MIHIA group indicates that their reservations about endorsing PE are based mainly on the number of administrative changes which would be required to implement the program.[29]

The Select Committee has recommended that TDHS implement ten to twelve PE pilots across the state in both urban and rural areas, using both MIHIA and non-MIHIA providers.[30] While the State Plan and administrative changes which will be required to enable implementation of PE are significant, they represent movement towards an integrated system of delivery of health care services to low-income Texans which is essential to attaining a more efficient use of public funds. Assuming a consensus that Texas should attempt to maximize the use of Medicaid and minimize the excessive costs of administration which are a byproduct of the balkanization of the health care delivery system, changes such as these can be seen as an inevitable part of achieving those goals. In fact, the most complex adjustments to the current perinatal network will be required in the process of implementing recommendations (5) and (6) below. The subsequent addition of PE will be relatively simple.

5) The Medicaid State Plan should be amended to allow for free-standing clinics, limited to maternal and child health reimbursement, as a provider type.

6) Free-standing clinics should offer prenatal medical care, risk assessment with appropriate referral, social and nutritional assessment and counseling, client education including family planning, postpartum care and case management services.[31]

Implementation of these recommendations will represent only a starting point for coordination of Medicaid with the MIHIA program. The interagency screening committee identified as objectives an aggressive client outreach and recruitment program and development of integrated eligibility programs which would also provide certain case management functions by making recipients aware of the existence of programs for which they are qualified. Since Medicaid is required to insure the availability of transportation to medical services for recipients, a coordination and expansion of the existing Medical Transportation

Program was recommended. Some mechanism for making prenatal vitamins available to Medicaid and MIHIA mothers (neither program currently provides these vitamins) should be devised. A systematic tracking system which could be used for case management, statistics and program management, and a program to raise physician awareness of the available services were among the committee's other recommendations for long-term activities.[32]

The steering committee suggested that the Medicaid expansion recommendations be adopted during the last two quarters of 1988, subject to "identification" of funds. The interagency group hopes to receive approval for the necessary State Plan amendments by August, 1988, and to make September 1, 1988 the effective date for adoption of the new coverage.[33] As of April, 1988, the U.S. House of Representatives' version of the Medicare Catastrophic Protection Act (HR 2470) which went to conference committee was reported to include an amendment which would mandate coverage of pregnant women and children up to 100% of poverty.[34] If such a proposal is included in the final version of the Act, any remaining barriers to implementation of the MOU recommendations will clearly be removed.

Cost Projections and Funding Methodology

The interagency report recommended two alternative approaches to claiming Medicaid reimbursement for services provided to the newly eligible population by providers who are also MIHIA providers.

The first strategy is referred to as "certification of funds." Under this scenario, TDH would make a quarterly estimate of the reimbursable services anticipated to be provided to Medicaid eligible MIHIA recipients, which TDHS would then include in its quarterly HCFA-25 estimate of Medicaid expenditures. The appropriate portion of the MIHIA budget would be certified by TDH as being available for the State's share of reimbursement. TDH would be responsible for reimbursing the providers for the Medicaid clients, and would continue to handle reimbursement for non-Medicaid MIHIA clients as well. Bills for MIHIA-Medicaid clients would be submitted to TDHS for review and audit.[35]

The second scenario, "transfer of funds", would also require the MIHIA program to provide TDHS with estimate of utilization of services by the newly Medicaid eligible clients. In this case, MIHIA providers would be instructed to bill TDHS directly for services provided to Medicaid recipients. TDHS would inform TDH of the cost of services to MIHIA recipients, and TDH would transfer from its budget (to TDHS) the state share of the costs.[36]

The second scenario seems more feasible. Given the complexity of Medicaid billings, it would be awkward and inefficient for the MIHIA program to have to master and to administer Medicaid reimbursement at the same time that it manages its own different reimbursement system. Of course, not all claims for newly eligible women and infants will be processed through the MIHIA program, since the program is not broad enough to serve as a gatekeeper for all the potentially eligible mothers as yet.

Widely varying estimates of the size of the uninsured (by Medicaid or private carrier) population of women with incomes less than 100% of poverty have been a major source of controversy in discussions over implementation of H.B. 1847. Specifically, TDH projected that there are about 105,000 births annually to such women in Texas. The estimate favored by TDHS staff was substantially smaller, at approximately 80,000.[37] Since the population in question has traditionally been under-served in the general area of human services, neither agency has had an opportunity to develop a clear profile for these potentially eligible people. The most current available census data were gathered in 1980 (and reflects 1979 incomes), so the margin of error may be substantial in projections of the number of women of reproductive age under 100% of poverty. Moreover, in addition to the size of that population, estimates must be made both of the number who have some other form of insurance (though not all of these will have coverage for maternity services), and of the number who will participate. The estimates which were used in developing the MOU and which were also presented to the Select Committee are described below.

In its most recent presentation to the Select Committee, TDHS projected that in 1989 there will be 36,640 births to women under poverty who are not currently covered by Medicaid, and that of these births, 15,404 would be paid for by Medicaid under the expanded eligibility. A summary of the projections presented to the committee is provided in Table 3.1. These projections reflect the department's estimate of the number of births under poverty being approximately 80,000 (44,110 + 36,640).[38]

Table 3.1
TDHS Projected Additional Costs
Due to Eligibility Expansions

	FY 1989	FY 1990	FY 1991
# Births to Women Under 100% FPL,w/o Medicaid	36,640	36,825	36,825
Projected Participation	60%	70%	80%
Births to Participants	21,984	25,778	29,460
Less Those Over Resource Limits	21,544	25,262	28,8717
Less Those with Private Insurance	15,404	18,062	20,643
# Births to Women under Current Eligibility Rules	44,110	44,325	44,325
Total Medicaid Births under Expansion	59,514	62,387	64,968
Estimated Total Costs*	$73,208,417	89,471,897	107,514,474
Estimated State's Share	$30,404,583	37,071,975	44,513,524
Addl. Costs for Enhanced Services to High Risk**	$2,547,199	2,819,892	3,092,477

State's Share of High Risk Costs	$1,043,333	1,115,267	1,174,213

* Includes costs of infant care up to age one.
** Estimated 40% of participants are high risk.

Source: Texas Dept. of Human Services, Budget and Analysis Division, presentation by Bryan Packard to Select Committee on Medicaid and Family Services, March 30, 1988.

The estimates proposed by TDH were based in part on a study which was commissioned by the department and conducted in the fall of 1986. The Texas OB Survey was designed to provide TDH with estimates of the unmet need for prenatal and maternity services in the state. The study projected that 58,320 Texas women with incomes less than poverty and with no third party coverage would give birth in 1987.[39] However, when the study distinguished between need for prenatal care and need for delivery, the delivery level was somewhat lower at 55,447, and the lower end of the 95% confidence interval for this estimate was 48,535. The authors also projected an additional 19,568 uninsured births to women between 100% and 200% of poverty.[40] TDHS estimated that there will be over 68,000 births to women between 100% and only 185% of poverty in 1988; however, this figure includes all women not covered by either Medicaid or MIHIA, and therefore includes a substantial number who have private insurance, which may account for the substantial difference between these two estimates.[41]

The American Hospital Association published in 1987 a lengthy report of recommendations and strategies for expansion of Medicaid eligibility at the state level, emphasizing especially the options created by

OBRA 1986. Included in the report are formulas for rough calculations of the costs of various expansions, and tabular data on all 50 states for use in calculating individual estimates. The AHA formula takes (1) an estimate of the number of women of reproductive age in Texas who are not served under the current Medicaid program. This number is reduced by the number of women under poverty who have private insurance (2), which is estimated to be 30% of such women. This would seem to be a reasonably accurate reduction; the 1985 Special Texas Census found that only 31.7% of Texans under poverty have private health insurance of any kind.[42] The resulting figure (3) is multiplied by (4) an adjusted fertility rate which was arrived at by adjusting the state fertility rate for the general population upwards by 12%, the percentage by which the birth rate of the national Medicaid population exceeds that of the general population. This product (5) is then multiplied by the projected utilization rate (6). The Congressional Budget Office estimates that 90% of eligible women will enroll; however, for purposes of this illustration, the TDHS estimate of 60% participation has been used. The resulting figure (7) is an estimate of the number of births to women under poverty with no other coverage than Medicaid.

AHA adds to the number calculated above another estimate of the costs of secondary coverage by Medicaid of births to women with another primary insurer. The insured portion of the non-Medicaid population (8) is estimated to give birth at the same rate, and of these births (9) approximately 25% of the costs are thought by the CBO to be borne by Medicaid (interestingly, CBO projects a 60% utilization rate for the double-coverage population). The resulting figure (10) is added to the first total to yield the final estimate of 16,650 additional covered births.[43] The entire calculation is illustrated below in Table 3.2.

Table 3.2:
AHA Projections of Additional Texas Births Under Medicaid Expansion

(1) 456,786 - (2) 178,798 = (3) 277,988
x (4) 0.086 = (5) 23,906.97
x (6) 0.60 = (7) 14,344.18

(8) 178,798 x 0.086 = (9) 15,376.63
x 0.60 = 9,225.98
x 0.25 = (10) 2,306.49

14,344 + 2,306 = 16,650

Source: Adapted from American Hospital Association, Medicaid Options: State Opportunities and Strategies for Expanding Eligibility (Chicago, 1987), pp. 60-63.

Given all the unknown factors involved in the projections, it is interesting that the AHA ball-park figure is this close to the TDHS estimate of 15,404. The interagency work groups apparently agreed that the TDHS estimates, though uncertain, were the best available. TDHS estimates that the unit cost for prenatal care, delivery and postpartum care of the mother plus infant care up to age one for her baby will be $4,310 (this does not include transportation, drugs, and other associated costs).[44] At this individual rate, the additional 1,246 eligible births indicated by the AHA projection would result increase the overall cost of the program by just over $5 million.

Table 3.3
TDHS,TDH and AHA Projections of Births at 100%, 185% and 200% Poverty (1989)

	Percent of Poverty		
	100%	**185%**	**200%**
TDHS: total without Medicaid	36,640	94,430	----
TDHS: adjusted for private insurance (28.5%) & excess resources (2%)	26,930	----	----
TDH: total with no third party payor	58,320	----	77,888
AHA: total with no third party payor	27,751	----	----

Sources: TDHS: Texas Department of Human Services, Budget and Data Analysis Division, "Number of Births to Women with Income Below 185% of Poverty Not Receiving Medicaid or MIHIA Services," February 17, 1988. (Handouts presented to select Committee on Medicaid and Family Services.)
AHA: Adapted from American Hospital Association, Medicaid Options: State Opportunities and Strategies for Expanding Eligibility (Chicago, 1987), pp. 60-63.

It is reasonable to expect that TDHS is in a far better position to project the effects of eligibility expansions than is any other entity. The difficulty experienced in arriving at and agreeing upon estimates illustrates one fundamental characteristic of Medicaid which is most troublesome to policy makers; that is, that even though it is easy to illustrate that too limited a Medicaid program results in the waste of resources, a reversal of that tradition requires the acceptance of a degree of uncertainty about utilization patterns and overall costs which is unprecedented in Texas' political experience.

But the case for improving Medicaid coverage of obstetrical services is especially compelling, since there is little question but that the services are ultimately going to be provided regardless of whether Medicaid coverage is available. There can also be little question but that those services are supported by state and local taxes. In short, a strong argument for effective prenatal care and coverage of maternity services can be made on purely economic grounds, setting aside any ethical considerations. This overwhelming economic evidence will no doubt insure that the first and most politically palatable expansions of Medicaid in Texas will be in maternal and child health.

As of this writing, adoption of the coverage of pregnant women and of children up to age one seems imminent. Texas has an opportunity with the adoption of eligibility for pregnant women under poverty to continue movement in the direction initiated by the Indigent Health Care Act; that is, towards the institution of a comprehensive, coordinated network of health care for the poor. Integrated eligibility, case management, free standing clinic services, and utilization of the expertise already acquired through MIHIA's experience are all components which have the potential to introduce a degree of coordination between city, county, state, federal and private sector efforts.

Realization of this potential will require a high degree of cooperation among the state agencies involved and the affected provider groups. THDS must work with HCFA to gain approval of all needed changes in the State Plan, and the agency bears the immediate responsibility for any sort of error penalties or disallowances arising from new programs. TDH has a legislative mandate to implement the Indigent Health Care Act and an understandable interest in the survival of the MIHIA network. Finally, hospitals and physicians are concerned about adequate reimbursement and possible limits on participation. Some sort of extra-agency executive oversight of the coordination process could expedite the process, but only if the overseeing body has expertise in the health care delivery area, adequate staffing and real authority. Though implementation of coverage of pregnant women and children may be inevitable, the approach to implementation is still open to question. At best, Texas should achieve substantial savings on uncompensated deliveries; at a minimum, the state should develop enough coordination in the delivery of health care services to indigent women and children to make it possible to estimate with some accuracy the true costs of service to this population.

Notes

1. Texas Department of Health, MIHIA Contracts, December 12, 1987. (Computer Printout.)

2. Testimony of C.E. Gibbs, M.D., Member MIHIA Advisory Committee, before Select Committee on Medicaid and Family Services, State Senate of Texas, February 11, 1988.

3. Texas Department of Human Services, Budget and Data Analysis Division, "Number of Births to Women with Income Below 100% of Poverty Not Receiving Medicaid or MIHIA Services," February 17, 1988. (Handouts presented to select Committee on Medicaid and Family Services.)

4. Texas Department of Health, MIHIA Contracts, December 12, 1987. (Computer Printout.)

5. TEX. REV. CIV. STAT. ANN. art 4447y, sec. 11 (Vernon 1976).

6. Paul A. Buescher, "Source of Prenatal Care and Infant Birthweight: the Case of a North Carolina County," SCHS Studies, no. 39 (March 1986), p. 5.

7. J.A. Lennie, "Low-Birth-Weight Rate Reduced by the Obstetrical Access Project," Health Care Financing Review, no. 8 (1987), pp. 83-86.

8. Paul A. Buescher, "Source of Prenatal Care and Infant Birthweight: the Case of a North Carolina County," SCHS Studies, no. 39 (March 1986), p. 6.

9. U.S. Department of Health and Human Services, Program Memorandum, Medicaid State Agencies, HCFA-Pub. 17, Transmittal No. 86-15, August 1986.

10. Ibid.

11. Ibid.

12. Telephone interview, Barbara Alexander, R.N., M.N., Department Head, Department of Obstetrics and Gynecology- High Risk Care, South Carolina Health and Human Services Financing Commission, Columbus, South Carolina, July 23, 1987.

13. Telephone interview with Ken Kamis, Director of Division of Primary Care, South Carolina Health and Human Services Financing Commission, Columbus, South Carolina, July 27, 1987.

14. National Health Care Campaign, Facing Facts: A Statistical Profile of Health Care in Texas, Washington, D.C., December, 1986, p. HC-16.

15. Department of Health Administration, Department of Epidemiology and Biostatistics, School of Public Health, University of South Carolina, Evaluation of the South Carolina Medicaid High Risk Channeling Project, (Columbia, October 1987), pp. 64-66.

16. Ibid, p. 56.

17. Telephone interview with Ann Wolff, Chief of Maternal and Child Health section, North Carolina Department of Human Services, Raleigh, July 21, 1987.

18. North Carolina Division of Medical Assistance, Operational Manual for Maternity Care Coordinator, Raleigh, n.d., p. II1-II2.

19. Telephone interview with Dennis Williams, Assistant Director of Medical Policy and Utilization Control, Division of Medical Assistance, North Carolina Department of Human Services, Raleigh, July 22, 1987.

20. Telephone interview with Dennis Williams, N.C. Dept. of Human Services, July 22, 1987.

21. Sara Rosenbaum, Director of Health Division, Children's Defense Fund, " Opportunities for Expanding the Scope of Indigent Health Activities in Texas That Can Be Financed as Medicaid Expenditures", December 3, 1986, p.7.(Memorandum.)

22. Interview with Lynn Hudson, R.N., N.P., Nurse Consultant, Bureau of Maternal and Child Health, Texas Department of Health, Austin, July 29, 1987.

23. TEX. REV. CIV. STAT. ANN. art 4447y, sec. 11 (Vernon 1976).

24. Texas Departments of Health and Human Services, " Maternal and Infant Health Care for Low-Income Texans: Memorandum of Understanding - A Final Report to the Commissioners," Austin, March 1988, p. 8.

25. Texas Legislature, Senate Select Committee on Medicaid and Family Services, "Draft Recommendations," (presented in Austin at March 30, 1988 meeting) p. 5.

26. Ibid., p. 9.

27. Ibid., p. 9-10.

28. P.L. 99-507, section 9407.

29. Texas Departments of Health and Human Services, " Maternal and Infant Health Care for Low-Income Texans: Memorandum of Understanding - A Final Report to the Commissioners," Austin, March 1988, pp. 10-12.

30. Texas Legislature, Senate Select Committee on Medicaid and Family Services, "Draft Recommendations," (presented in Austin at March 30, 1988 meeting) p. 3.

31. Texas Departments of Health and Human Services, " Maternal and Infant Health Care for Low-Income Texans: Memorandum of Understanding - A Final Report to the Commissioners," Austin, March 1988, pp. 17-19.

32. Ibid., pp. 22-25.

33. Ibid., pp. 25-26.

34. "Proposal Would Make More Mothers-To-Be Eligible for Medicaid," El Paso Times, April 8, 1988, sec. B, p. 2.

35. Texas Departments of Health and Human Services, " Maternal and Infant Health Care for Low-Income Texans: Memorandum of Understanding - A Final Report to the Commissioners," Austin, March 1988, p. 21.

36. Ibid.

37. Interview with Ernest Schmid, Director Indigent Health Care Program, Texas Department of Human Services, Austin, November 11, 1988.

38. Texas Department of Human Services, Budget and Data Analysis Division, Presentation by Bryan Packard to Select Committee on Medicaid and Family Services, March 30, 1988.

39. Public Policy Resources Laboratory, Texas A & M University, "Texas OB Survey: Determining the Need for Maternity Services in Texas - County Projections," (Submitted to Texas Department of Health, May 22, 1987), p. 6.

40. Public Policy Resources Laboratory, Texas A & M University, "Texas OB Survey: Determining the Need for Maternity Services in Texas," (Submitted to Texas Department of Health, March 23, 1987), p. 17.

41. Texas Department of Human Services, Budget and Data Analysis Division, "Number of Births to Women with Income Below 185% of Poverty Not Receiving Medicaid or MIHIA Services," February 17, 1988. (Handouts presented to select Committee on Medicaid and Family Services.)

42. Texas Department of Human Services, Budget and Planning Division, "1985 Special Texas Census: Summary of Selected Findings," Austin, October 15, 1986. (Photocopied.)

43. Irene Fraser, Phd., _Medicaid Options: State Opportunities and Strategies for Expanding Eligibility_, (Chicago: American Hospital Association, 1987), pp. 41, 60-63, 122.

44. Texas Department of Human Services, Budget and Data Analysis Division, Presentation by Bryan Packard to Select Committee on Medicaid and Family Services, March 30, 1988.

Chapter Four
Expanding Medicaid Coverage of MHMR Services

The discussion of expansions of various types of services in the mental health and mental retardation areas provides insight into some of the most troublesome cost control problems presented by Medicaid. Two cases are discussed briefly; the addition of optional mental health services and the current controversy over reimbursement of ICF-MRs. Neither of these programs is under formal consideration for reform in the immediate future. They are included in this report because they illustrate well a number of policy issues which are fundamental to the subject of Medicaid expansion.

Mental Health Services

With legal pressure on the state to make improvements in the MHMR system, potential new sources of funding are of particular interest. Texas has the option of adding several types of mental health coverage to the Medicaid program. Specifically, Texas could choose to add the optional service of coverage of services in "institutions for mental diseases" (IMDs: includes psychiatric hospitals) for Medicaid eligible persons under age 22 or over age 65. By adding diagnostic, screening and rehabilitation services, the state might be able to cover services currently provided in state mental health outreach centers and community MHMR clinics.

These options have not been exercised in the past primarily because if low income users of mental health services can use Medicaid to pay for their care, they can take their Medicaid cards to any provider which meets state standards and is willing to accept Medicaid, and they may not necessarily choose state- or locally-funded facilities. In a worst case, an actual net loss to the state could result from such a shift in utilization patterns. This potential naturally exists with all Medicaid expansions; however, it is thought to be most serious in the mental health and mental retardation area because the general public perceives public sector services in this area to be less appealing than those the private sector offers. Federal judgments against the state hospital and state school systems have tended to reinforce this perception.

Background

These mental health options are not new. When the option to cover IMD services to those under age 21 was established by federal law in 1972, a Governor's Task Force was created to study the option, which was not implemented. Coverage of the population older than 65 in IMDs was actually offered between 1967 and 1975, and was discontinued because of additional costs to the state which resulted from shift to private providers. In 1978, TDHS contracted with a consultant firm to conduct a study of the costs of implementing both the over 65 and the under 22 coverage. The results of this study led the agency to conclude that expansion at that time entailed too much financial risk for the state, and no action was taken.[1]

The R.A.J. v. Miller lawsuit, which alleged that Texas state mental hospitals failed to provide adequate treatment in the least restrictive environment possible, was filed in 1974. The settlement of the suit in 1981 stimulated renewed interest in Medicaid as a source of funding for mental health services. One of the central stipulations of the settlement was that the state would reduce patient-staff ratios in state hospitals; the state has chosen to achieve this goal principally via deinstitutionalization of inpatients to community homes, rather than through direct enhancement of staffing levels. The subsequent finding in 1984 by the R.A.J. review panel that the state was not in compliance with some terms of the settlement led to the establishment of a Legislative Oversight Committee on Mental Health and Mental Retardation, which requested in 1985 another study of Medicaid mental health expansions.

This study, which was produced jointly by the Texas Department of Mental Health and Mental Retardation (TDMHMR) and TDHS, stressed the difficulty in estimating the potential demand for mental health services and the consequent uncertainty surrounding cost estimates of adding the mental health services.[2] It was estimated that addition of IMD coverage for the over 65 population would have made about 80% of patients in that age group at that time eligible. A net savings to the state of $5.5 million was projected if SNF/ICF services were not included; but inclusion of the SNF/ICF services was projected to result in an increase in costs to the state of $4 million because of the degree of private sector participation in those services.[3] The agencies found that inpatient IMD coverage of the under 22 population would have covered 62% of that age group population in the state hospitals, and would cost the state and additional

$18.9 million because of the great number of young people in private sector IMDs who would be covered.[4] The study concluded that IMD services (including SNF/ICF) for the over 65 be implemented in the short term, and that a proposal for services to the under 22 population be developed for future implementation.[5]

Recent Analysis

No immediate action was taken on these recommendations. In July of 1987, the R.A.J. review panel once again found inadequate compliance by the state. In 1987 TDMHMR commissioned a study by an independent consultant of potential benefits or losses from adding the services mentioned above, looking also at the option of adding diagnostic, screening and rehabilitation services. The report detailed areas in which Medicaid requirements for mental health services may exceed the service levels now provided by Texas programs. The study also looked into specific mechanisms used by other states which moderate private sector participation in the program, and thus limit the shift of state dollars to the private sector. Significant findings of the study are summarized below, beginning with an explanation of the diagnostic, screening and rehabilitation (DSR) option.

Diagnostic, Screening and Rehabilitation Services

Texas communities are served by Community MHMR centers which provide services either directly or by contract in 137 counties. State Centers in El Paso, Laredo and the Rio Grande Valley also provide a wide range of mental health services. Since 1985, Community MHMR Centers have been required by state law to provide a number of core services. These services include crisis stabilization, contracted inpatient beds (for stabilization of acute psychiatric crises), multi-disciplinary assessment of acutely dysfunctional clients, family support programs, case management, psychosocial rehabilitation services, and medication related services. Subsumed under the last category are a number of services involved in the prescription of psychotropic drugs, including monitoring of medications by laboratory and physical examination, and ongoing education and therapy for clients using medication.[6] It is thought that many of the services provided in community clinics could be covered by Medicaid under the rubric of DSR services.

States offering mental health clinic services paid for under DSR have limited program costs by application of the same standards to public and private providers alike. For example, all Medicaid clinics may be required to submit to the state reports outlining immediate and long range goals, and projections of growth and of Medicaid utilization. Several states require that all clinic providers contract with the state to serve Medicaid clients. States also mandate staffing levels or require Medicaid clinics to remain open some minimum number of hours per week, and, in Colorado, Medicaid qualified clinics must serve all persons from the clinics' service area regardless of their ability to pay. Reimbursement levels are controlled through the use of maximum allowable fees for specific services.[7]

<u>Institutions for Mental Diseases</u>

Under federal rules, implementation of the over 65 option would require that the Medicaid agency (TDHS) maintain and review an individual plan of treatment for each IMD client. TDHS would also be required to demonstrate in annual progress reports to HCFA that Texas was "making satisfactory progress in developing and implementing a comprehensive mental health program."[8] Under regulations governing services to persons under 22, it is stipulated that inpatient psychiatric services must be provided in freestanding facilities, and not in psychiatric wards of general hospitals. A team of mental health professionals must monitor the care of each (under 22) patient. Each team must include either (1) a board-certified psychiatrist or (2) a doctorate level psychologist and a physician.[9] The report did not indicate to what extent existing staff levels could accommodate this requirement.

Other states have clearly shared Texas' need to assure that expansions of Medicaid coverage be as nearly budget-neutral as possible. Approaches taken by other states to contain program costs have included enhanced per diem reimbursement rates to IMD facilities with high percentages of Medicaid or indigent patients, disallowance of depreciation and interest on new beds, exclusion of chemical dependency services, and use of median costs in calculation of per diem rates. California (under a waiver) contracts only with enough facilities to insure access to all Medicaid patients within the greater of normal community travel time or 30 minutes. In Michigan, qualified Medicaid IMDs are required to accept involuntarily committed patients; in Colorado, all IMD clients must be referred by a community mental health authority.[10]

<u>Cost Estimates</u>

The study cautions in the case of each of the three options that there are no studies available of the demand for mental health services in Texas, and that all estimates are based on demand projections drawn from original data in other states. However, the report does make a set of cost projections for each option, including alternative scenarios based on different levels of private sector participation. Approaches to controlling program cost for each option are also included.

Implementation of DSR services is estimated to bring in reimbursement to TDMHMR and the community clinics of $25 to $30 million above the state's share if there is no private sector participation in the program. If the number of Medicaid eligible clients now being served by TDMHMR and the Community Centers were increased by 50%, and if that 50% were served by the private sector, the consultants estimate that the net benefit to the public sector programs would still be over $15 million. If private sector participation were to increase to 125% of the size of that current eligible population, the state match dollars going to pay for private care would then exceed the federal dollars coming in to TDMHMR and the Community Centers.[11]

To control program growth, the study recommends that all qualified providers be required to meet the same guidelines now applied to community MHMR centers pertaining to documentation, reporting, physical plant, financial condition, quality assurance, staff to client ratios, and staff qualifications. In order to participate, providers would have to submit to periodic audits regarding their compliance with these standards. In addition, it is suggested that providers be required to make services available to all chronically mentally ill persons in the service area regardless of ability to pay, and to prepare and submit annual projections of indigent care and utilization of public funds from all sources.[12]

Cost estimates for the over 65 option project a $15 million benefit to the state if there were no private sector participation. If every existing empty private sector bed (certified as freestanding psychiatric by TDMHMR) was filled with a Medicaid recipient, the net benefit to the state is estimated to still exceed $9 million. If the private sector filled 75% of existing capacity with Medicaid clients, the break-even point between state match and reimbursement returning to the state would be reached. If the private sector expanded capacity by 25% and devoted its entire capacity to Medicaid clients, the study projects a net loss to the state of $9 million.[13]

In the absence of any private sector participation, the under 22 option is projected to bring in $8-$9 million additional dollars to the state, and if all empty private sector beds were occupied by Medicaid clients, a net benefit to the state of $4-$5 million is projected. It is expected that the break-even point would be reached if the private sector filled 50% of existing beds with Medicaid clients, and that a net loss of $6-$8 million would result from 100% occupation of existing private sector beds by Medicaid clients.[14]

The proposals for cost control are quite similar for the two IMD options. The state is cautioned that limits on length of stay are likely to be punitive to the public sector facilities who will serve the bulk of chronic (long-term) clients. Other recommended approaches are basically the same as those proposed for the DSR option; that is, conservative reimbursement policies, universal licensure standards, and mandatory reporting and accounting requirements. Qualified provider hospitals could also, like DSR providers, be required to provide services to the chronically mentally ill population in the service area, regardless of ability to pay.

The analysis provided by the consultants did not attempt to associate the use of the approaches described above with the probability of any specific level of private sector participation in the programs; therefore no most-likely cost estimate was identified. The analysis does underscore the conflict between budget neutrality and open private sector participation in the Medicaid network. Further observations on this topic are deferred to the end of this chapter.

One topic not addressed by the study was the precise mechanism by which the state's share for these new services would be generated. Would TDMHMR commit to the Medicaid program (to TDHS) funds now appropriated directly to state hospitals, or granted to Community MHMR Centers? Implementation of optional mental health services would seem to be a fiscally sound move; however, from the perspective of each of the affected agencies, certain risks are involved. In effect, TDMHMR is required to relinquish a measure of control over certain funds, while TDHS must bear the ultimate responsibility for programs administered in large part by another agency. Thus, programs which require a coordinated effort between two state agencies must overcome not only logistical barriers but also political ones, particularly when the locus of control over a significant amount of state money is being manipulated.

The magnitude of the difficulty of such efforts has only begun to be demonstrated by the process of coordination of MIHIA and Medicaid. Movement towards a broader Medicaid program will inevitably necessitate ever greater degrees of cooperation between agencies, and it stands to reason that aggressive coordination of services will be needed to minimize duplications of effort. Another case study in the problems of interagency coordination and management of Medicaid program costs is provided by the short history of the TDMHMR Prospective Payment Program for ICF-MRs.

ICF-MRs and the PPP

There are three state agencies directly involved with the functioning of ICF-MRs, the community homes for the mentally retarded. Homes are certified and licensed by TDH. Policies and standards for the homes are initiated and developed by TDMHMR, and are subsequently adopted by the TDHS Board. The TDHS board sets Medicaid reimbursement rates for the facilities, and the agency itself is of course responsible for reimbursement for Medicaid clients. ICF-MR services are also provided in the setting of a number of State Schools. Services to Medicaid eligible clients in these facilities are supported by direct state appropriations, and reimbursement by Medicaid is made to the State Treasury.

A class action suit, Lelsz v. Kavanagh, was filed in 1974, alleging that state schools for the mentally retarded were providing inadequate care and were improperly institutionalizing clients. The ICF-MR program predates the settlement of that suit in

1983, but the mandatory deinstitutionalization of State School residents pursuant to that settlement has stimulated considerable growth in the number of facilities. In 1986 there were a total of 163 community based ICF-MRs receiving Medicaid reimbursement in Texas.[15] Though reimbursement of homes is considered inadequate by private providers, the number of homes has grown steadily, and reimbursement has repeatedly threatened to deplete appropriated funds. More than half of existing ICF-MR facilities are owned by five different owners; one group alone operates 40 six-bed homes.[16] According to the TAPP, over 97% of residents in private sector ICF-MRs are Medicaid recipients.[17]

The earliest ICF-MR facilities were converted nursing homes with 50 to 60 bed capacities. Maximum allowable size for the facilities has been reduced twice; first to 15 beds, and most recently to six beds per facility. These reductions have been made largely as a measure of cost control. Since the basis for rates has been the costs of larger facilities which may benefit from economies of scale, reducing the number of beds has limited the profitability of operation of ICF-MRs (at current reimbursement levels), slowed growth in the number of providers, and thereby limited the state's liability for Medicaid payments to ICF-MRs. The six bed limitation is also intended to encourage homes which are compatible with the goal of community based services. A special statewide zoning variance allows homes up to six beds to locate in areas where they might otherwise be prohibited by local zoning regulations.

In the wake of the Lelsz decision, however, it became necessary for the state to come up with some incentive to encourage ICF-MR growth in order to create homes for newly deinstitutionalized State School residents. TDMHMR considered making funds available to TDHS to raise reimbursement rates for the homes. Due to general apprehension that raising Medicaid rates to reflect true costs would result in a flood of new providers who would all have to be paid regardless of budget constraints, this option was rejected. The Prospective Payment Program (PPP) was created as a way to fund community homes while allowing the state to limit its liability to a fixed amount.[18]

The PPP does not fund Medicaid patients in ICF-MRs exclusively; funds also go to other providers such as Group Homes and Alternative Living Centers. The program now provides a payment of $55.60 per day per client (or $20,294 per annum) to the homes. Homes are now receiving this payment for about 400 clients in ICF-MRs who are also Medicaid recipients. Both the Texas Council of Community MHMR Centers and the Texas Association of Private Providers (an industry group representing private ICF-MR owners) have stated that the true cost of service in the six-bed homes is $80-$100 per day.[19] The 1988 Medicaid reimbursement rates for ICF-MRs are $57.32 for level I, $48.40 for level V and $59.05 for level VI homes,[20] so for clients also covered by PPP the daily rate is over $100, of which about 70% are state dollars. These rates are set in the TDHS nursing home program by applying inflationary and occupancy adjustments to a cost base derived from two-year old data.

In March of 1988, the Texas Attorney General announced that it was investigating the possibility that providers who were receiving both Medicaid reimbursement and PPP funding for the same clients might be in violation of federal regulations which prohibit any sort of supplementary payments to Medicaid providers for Medicaid services. In theory, the homes could legitimately receive supplementary payments only if the payments were used exclusively for services not covered by Medicaid. Officials at TDMHMR say that they have made this requirement clear to providers. Owners of homes have been quick to seize the opportunity provided by press coverage of the investigation to publicize the inadequacy of the Medicaid rates, and in doing so have apparently admitted that PPP funds were used to supplement Medicaid payments, after all.[21]

Texas Attorney General Jim Mattox has stated that investigation of the PPP thus far has indicated that funds are not being used for additional services. If the program is found to violate federal guidelines, he has said, providers might be required to return funds to the state. Statements from the attorney general's office left open the possibility that criminal charges may be filed as a result of the investigation.[22] At this writing, TDMHMR has announced that it will not offer to provide PPP funding to any new participant homes until the attorney general's investigation has been completed. At least two NFP homes which had planned to open in April of 1988 have suspended activity because management does not believe that the homes can be operated without the PPP funds.[23]

The attorney general's office has a responsibility to monitor Medicaid fraud and abuse. If

MHMR's policy violates Medicaid regulations it is in the state's interest that the violation be detected early in order to limit the state's liability for penalties which may be imposed by HCFA. It is surprising that the attorney general's office has framed the problem as an investigation of the providers themselves, since the policy was developed and promoted by the state agencies involved. Attorney General Mattox has expressed concern that the state may have to assume all of the financial liability if it should be determined that the PPP-Medicaid combination does constitute fraud (however, no precise indication of what that liability might consist was given).[24] A degree of irony would accompany a determination of fraud, given that the "double-dipping" funding of the affected homes was devised as a way to limit program costs. It seems unlikely that the practice could be considered fraud, since the term assumes a deliberate intent to obtain funding through misrepresentation. Furthermore, if it can be established that the rates being paid by Medicaid are indeed inadequate, the State would be out of compliance with the Boren Amendment, which requires states to set Medicaid rates which are adequate to cover the costs of services at a level which will conform with all state and federal regulations.

Problems: Interagency Cooperation and the Role of Private Sector Providers

These scenarios from the mental health area underscore several points. First, the existence of a need for interagency cooperation in the process of making a transition from state funding of a program to Medicaid funding seems to increase the difficulty of the process by a substantial magnitude. Where a legislative mandate for coordination exists, oversight of interagency task forces by a person or persons not affiliated with either agency might expedite problem-solving between the agencies. This approach presumes the availability of persons with adequate expertise to balance the sometimes incongruent interests of the affected agencies along with the larger state program goals. Such persons are very likely in short supply and their time may be limited, expensive, or both. Whatever the solution, it would seem that some mechanism or incentive for agencies to place state goals ahead of agency interests is missing in the process.

The cost-benefit estimates of adding optional mental health services to the Medicaid State Plan provided by both the 1985 TDMHMR-TDHS study and the recent consultants' report indicate a high degree of confidence that considerable savings of state money could result from such changes. What is also made clear is that the changes will only result in direct savings to the state to the extent to which private sector participation in the programs can be limited. However, overt acknowledgement of this fact is not politically acceptable, because of an unarticulated but potent acceptance that the primacy of free enterprise should not be impinged upon, even in the arena of indigent health care. It is probably necessary to accept this state of affairs as a bit of political reality. However, it is unfortunate that the assumption that private sector participation should not be limited cannot be examined in a more explicit fashion. Acceptance of unlimited private sector participation, or the characterization of efforts to limit such participation as being unfair, are simply incompatible with a commitment to budget neutrality. Those who support open access to the Medicaid market must be willing to fund, by whatever means necessary, the additional costs to the state which would result.

The approaches used by other states to limit private participation are not truly exclusionary in most cases. As noted, simply requiring of all providers the same standards of licensure and reporting normally applied to public entities is often adequate to discourage prospective private providers. This practice reflects a defendable adherence to the standards of accountability which are expected in the public sector. Reimbursement levels are often used as engineering tools in these programs; when less participation is desired, reimbursement is less generous, and when growth is desired the rates are increased. When rates are so low that access to services is threatened for Medicaid recipients, providers' complaints of inadequacy of payment may well be justified. Still, there is a philosophical (as opposed to purely economic) basis for the use of methodologies which try to limit payments to direct costs. These policies reflect a belief that programs designed to serve impoverished or disadvantaged persons should not make other people rich in the process.

This last proposition, the idea that Medicaid does not necessarily need to be profitable, is clearly at odds with the "free enterprise" attitude mentioned above. The fact that there is little public dialogue and thus little coherent public policy direction on the question suggests that the tension between these incompatible values will continue to figure heavily in the choices made in Medicaid policy in Texas.

Notes

1. Texas Department of Human Services and Texas Department of Mental Health and Mental Retardation, Extending Medicaid to Cover Mental Health Services: A Report to the Lieutenant Governor, (Austin, March 15, 1985), p. I-1.

2. Ibid., p. 2.

3. Ibid., p. IV-6.

4. Ibid., p. IV-7.

5. Ibid., pp. VI 1-VI 2.

6. TEX. REV. CIV. STAT. ANN. art. 5547-204, sec. 4.03.

7. Texas Department of Mental Health and Mental Retardation, "Option: Diagnostic,Screening and Rehabilitation," (Draft of report by Touche Ross, Austin, 1987),pp. 37-39.

8. Texas Department of Mental Health and Mental Retardation, "Medicaid Optional Services: Institutes for Mental Diseases for Patients Over 65," (Draft of report by Touche Ross, Austin, 1987), pp. 45-46.

9. Texas Department of Mental Health and Mental Retardation, "Medicaid Optional Service: Inpatient Psychiatric Under 22," (Draft of report by Touche Ross, Austin, 1987), pp. 58-59.

10. Texas Department of Mental Health and Mental Retardation, "Medicaid Optional Services: Institutes for Mental Diseases for Patients Over 65," (Draft of report by Touche Ross, Austin, 1987), pp. 47-49.

11. Texas Department of Mental Health and Mental Retardation, "Option: Diagnostic,Screening and Rehabilitation," (Draft of report by Touche Ross, Austin, 1987),p. 44.

12. Ibid., pp. 40-43.

13. Texas Department of Mental Health and Mental Retardation, "Medicaid Optional Services: Institutes for Mental Diseases for Patients Over 65," (Draft of

report by Touche Ross, Austin, 1987), pp. 54-57.

14. Texas Department of Mental Health and Mental Retardation, "Medicaid Optional Service: Inpatient Psychiatric Under 22," (Draft of report by Touche Ross, Austin, 1987), pp. 66,69.

15. Texas Department of Human Services, "Reimbursement Rates for CY 1988 for Community Based Intermediate Care Facilities for the Mentally Retarded," (Memorandum regarding agenda item no. 5, Texas Board of Human Services meeting, Austin, December 17, 1987).

16. "State Inquiry Targets Homes for the Retarded," Austin American-Statesman, March 18, 1988, p. B-8.

17. Testimony of Richard Johnson, Texas Association of Private Providers, before Texas Board of Human Services (agenda item no. 5), Austin, December 17, 1987.

18. Telephone Interview with Spencer McClure, Executive Director, Texas Council of Community MHMR Centers, Austin, December 14, 1987.

19. "State Inquiry Targets Homes for the Retarded," Austin American-Statesman, March 18, 1988, p. B-1.

20. Texas Department of Human Services, "Reimbursement Rates for CY 1988 for Community Based Intermediate Care Facilities for the Mentally Retarded," (Memorandum regarding agenda item no. 5, Texas Board of Human Services meeting, Austin, December 17, 1987).

21. "State Inquiry Targets Homes for the Retarded," Austin American-Statesman, March 18, 1988, sec. B, pp. 1,8.

22. "Homes May Be Told to Return Medicaid Funds," Austin American-Statesman, March 30, 1988, sec. B, p. 3.

23. "Funds Cut to Homes for the Retarded," Austin American-Statesman, April 6, 1988, sec. B pp. 1, 8.

24. "Homes May Be Told to Return Medicaid Funds," Austin American-Statesman, March 30, 1988, sec. B, p. 3.

Chapter Five
Prospective Payment of Inpatient Hospitalization Costs Under Medicaid in Texas

There are a number of reasons to consider changes in hospital reimbursement as part of a Medicaid expansion plan. The survival of the hospital industry is obviously critical if we are to be able to provide health care services to the poor at a reasonable cost. Making thousands more Texans eligible for Medicaid will be of little value if reimbursement standards are so inadequate that more and more hospitals choose not to accept Medicaid patients. If rural hospitals or hospitals which serve a largely indigent population are forced to close their doors, the cost of providing care to the population which Texas has made a legal commitment to serve can be expected to increase dramatically. Aside from these considerations, the chances of an expansion of funding and eligibility actually being implemented will be greatly enhanced by the support of the hospitals of Texas for the plan.

Given the above rationale, this chapter will briefly outline the evolution of the current prospective payment system, particularly as it illustrates issues in reimbursement which are of ongoing concern to Texas hospitals. Some issues which have not yet been addressed by the system will also be discussed, along with recommendations for changes in the system.

The Peer Group System

On September 1, 1986 TDHS began reimbursing hospitals for inpatient services under a new Texas based Diagnosis Related Group (DRG) system. Under this system, each hospital receiving Medicaid reimbursement was placed into one of three "Peer Group" classifications: Children's hospitals, Teaching hospitals or Other Hospitals. Each of the three peer groups was assigned a Standard Dollar Amount (SDA); $2,511.73 for children's hospitals, $1,911.26 for teaching hospitals and $1,541.33 for other hospitals. The DRG classification designations used by Medicare were adopted for the program, but the relative weights and the average lengths of stay assigned to those DRGs were developed specifically for the Texas Medicaid system based on cost report data from 1985.[1]

Under the DRG system, payment of a hospital claim proceeds as follows. When a patient is dismissed or has exhausted his 30 days of eligibility, the hospital can bill Medicaid. The patient stay must be assigned a specific DRG by the hospital, using the same software program which assigns Medicare patients to DRGs. The amount paid to the provider is the DRG relative weight multiplied by the hospital's SDA (assuming that the patient was eligible for his entire stay). No adjustments are made for "outliers"; that is, for stays which require an unusually high intensity of services, or for unusually long stays. There are no urban versus rural distinctions, nor is there any other type of hospital specific adjustment to the payment.[2]

Texas specific relative weights for the DRGs were calculated by dividing the average of all paid claims for a given DRG in 1985 by the average of payments for all DRGs in 1985. Where fewer than ten claims had been submitted to Medicaid for a given DRG in 1985, the Medicare relative weight was used. The average length of stay for a DRG was the calculated mean stay for that DRG in 1985. The computation of the three SDAs is not explained here because, unlike the relative weight and average length of stay methodologies, it is no longer used.[3]

Reactions to Peer Group Methodology

Reaction by hospitals to the new system was immediate and negative. The Texas Hospital Association (THA) established a Technical Advisory Group (TAG) to work with the TDHS Health Care Services staff on revisions to the DRG system even before the original system was implemented. Hospitals found much about the new system which they did not like; however, discussion of many of those perceived problems which were not rectified under the revised DRG system is reserved for later in this chapter.

The most glaring problem was the three peer group SDA system. Although the intention of the groupings was to treat hospitals with like costs in a like fashion, analysis of the costs of those hospitals revealed an enormous range of costs within each category. In fact, in the "other" hospitals category, the SDA of $1,541 took in 439 hospitals with a range in case mix adjusted cost per case from as low as $356.96 to as high as $5,014.83. The ranges in the teaching and children's hospital groups were ameliorated somewhat by the fact that they contained considerably fewer (35 and 5, respectively) hospitals, but they had the same effect of producing "winners" and "losers" under the new system.[4]

The Creation of the PDI System

The reaction of THA to the perceived inequity of the original DRG system was strong enough that by the end of September of 1986, the same month in which prospective reimbursement had begun, TDHS had agreed to accept an alternative peer grouping methodology which was proposed by THA. This new system assigns each hospital to a payment division increment (PDI) according to the average Medicaid payment per case for that hospital in the base year of 1985. Each increment represents $100, so that a hospital in PDI seven would have had an average cost in 1985 between $600 and $700. Any PDI which contains fewer than ten observations (hospitals) is assigned to the next higher category which does contain 10 or more hospitals. The new system was implemented on April 1, 1987.[5]

One significant problem remained with the PDI system; any hospital with a low claim count, but most particularly small or rural hospitals, faced prohibitively low reimbursement if it was unlucky enough to have had relatively low-cost Medicaid clients in the base year of 1985. And, since the system is re-based only every three years, these providers would have had to live with the consequences of their poor fortune for some time to come. Naturally this problem contributed to a lack of consensus among THA members regarding the desirability of the new PDI system.

To remedy this situation, the TDHS board approved in July of 1987 a rule change which would make $1,200 the minimum SDA under the system. This change is expected to benefit between 125 to 157[6] hospitals, some of which had SDAs as low as $357 under the original PDI structure. The new minimum took effect

November 1, 1987, and is expected to cost between $3 and $4 million.[7]

Two other adjustments to the PDI system have been made by TDHS. The first is the inclusion of return on equity as an allowable cost in the calculation of hospital costs in the base year. Hospitals had complained that the exclusion of return on equity contributed to underestimation of true costs for providers.[8] The rationale for exclusion had been that Medicaid was not intended to be a source of profit for hospitals. However, this philosophy is somewhat at odds with one of the purposes of DRG systems; namely, to create incentives for hospitals to cut costs by guaranteeing the full DRG payment even when costs are below the payment level.

The other major change has been the creation of an appeals process for the prospective payment system. Parkland Hospital in Dallas filed suit early in 1987 to attempt to enjoin TDHS from implementing the PDI system. An injunction did not result; however, negotiations between Parkland and TDHS led to the development of the appeals process. Under the process which went into effect on September 22, 1987, a hospital may request review of mathematical, mechanical or data entry errors in computation of base year data, or errors in any later adjustments to the base year claims data.[9]

<u>PDI Methodology</u>

An understanding of the basics of the system used in assigning hospitals to PDIs is useful in understanding some of the remaining unresolved issues in prospective payment. A brief explanation of the methodology is provided below.

Hospitals are assigned to PDIs according to a value referred to as the Hospital Specific Standard Dollar Amount. Several steps are involved in arriving at this figure. First, a Case Mix Index (CMI) value is calculated from base year data, which is simply the average of all of the DRG relative weights in the hospital's base year file. The Average Dollars Paid (ADP) on a Medicaid claim for the hospital in the base year is calculated by dividing the total amount paid by Medicaid and other insurance for Medicaid patients by the total number of patient stays. The Average Dollars Paid is then divided by the Case Mix Index to yield Standardized Dollars per Case. This figure is then increased for inflation by 10.88% and reduced by 10% to reflect an across the board cut in funding first made in 1986 due to state budget constraints. The result is the Hospital Specific Standard Dollar Amount (HSSDA).

$$(ADP/CMI)x(1.1088)x(0.9)=HSSDA$$

This last figure is the basis for assignment to a PDI. Assuming that the PDI contains 10 or more providers, the Standard Dollar Amount for all hospitals in that particular PDI is calculated as follows. First, each provider's HSSDA is multiplied by the total number of stays in its base year data. The average (mean) of these products for all hospitals in the PDI becomes the SDA for reimbursement of that set of providers.[10]

Unresolved Issues:

Cost vs. Claims Paid

One of the changes in the prospective payment system (PPS) which has been advocated by THA involves the data base used for the calculations outlined above. Those calculations are based on the dollar amounts of claims actually paid, as opposed to recorded costs for a stay. There are any number of instances in which the paid amount is less than the recorded cost. One example is the costs of care for patients who stay in the hospital longer than the 30 day maximum for which Texas Medicaid will pay. The Association recommends changing to a cost based calculation of SDAs.[11]

Cost Outliers

One other thing which should be pointed out about the claims paid values is that, as noted in the methodology description, the figures include other third party ("other insurance") payments for Medicaid eligible patients. TDHS chose to include these payments, which it contends are typically more generous than Medicaid reimbursement, as a way to make the data base more generous in compensation for some of the areas in which the methodology is more parsimonious.[12]

TDHS has held that because the data base includes high cost claims on Medicaid stays which were paid by third parties, there is no need for a special methodology to compensate hospitals for extraordinarily expensive cases referred to as "cost outliers". DRG reimbursement under Medicare does provide some coverage of cost outliers. The THA Technical Advisory Group points out that the database also includes very low cost claims paid, such as claims paid for stays for which the patient was not eligible for the entire period of hospitalization. THA holds that as a result there is no effective upward skew in the relative weights as alleged by TDHS, and a methodology for cost outliers needs to be created.[13]

30 Day Length of Stay and Per Diem Pricing

The 30-day limit per spell of illness on payments for inpatient hospital stays mentioned above is itself a major issue in the PPS. A patient is covered for up to 30 days of hospitalization, which may be used in either a single or in multiple visits. After his 30 days are exhausted, he must remain unhospitalized for 60 consecutive days before he again is eligible for another 30 days of coverage. If a patient does not have as many remaining eligible days as the actual length of his stay, the hospital is reimbursed on a per diem basis according to the following formula:

[(DRG rel. wt.xSDA)/DRG ALOS]x[# Days Eligible].

THA has made the strong point that because the SDAs and the DRG relative weights were both calculated using only allowable eligible days (claims paid), the 30-day limit is already reflected in those rates for all reimbursements. It is the contention of the Association that the per diem reimbursement amounts to a "double hit". On this basis, THA recommends that hospitals should be paid the full DRG amount if the patient had any eligible days at all remaining during the stay.[14]

Since there are no provisions under Texas' Medicaid PPS for outliers, a hospital can expect to receive no reimbursement whatsoever for care provided beyond the 30 day limit. Under the federal Medicare PPS, length-of-stay outliers are reimbursed at a limited rate after they exceed the average length of stay for that DRG by the lesser of 20 days or 1.94 standard deviations. THA recommends the establishment of a like provision under the Medicaid PPS to protect hospitals from the burden of uncompensated stays of an extraordinary length.

Frequency of Re-basing

It was noted previously that relative weights for DRGs, Hospital Specific Standard Dollar Amounts and the SDAs for each Payment Division Increment are all derived from data in annual Medicaid Cost Reports. More specifically, current rates are derived from 1985 cost reports and then adjusted for inflation. Under current regulation the entire system is to be recalculated every three years. Hospitals are concerned that the length of this period will create a disincentive for high-volume Medicaid providers to make capital improvements, since the reimbursement structure may not recognize new costs for several years. Likewise, increased expenses for medical education could be penalized under the existing system.[15]

The Medicare PPS is re-based annually. The THA advocates that Texas follow suit for Medicaid. Since the cost reports from which rates are derived are filed annually, this change would be feasible, although administrative costs would no doubt be greater for annual re-basing.

Data Base Problems: Nominal Charge and Low-Volume Providers

One of the assumptions upon which the equity of the Medicare PPS system relies is the concept of "leveling"; that is, that a hospital which sustains a loss on a DRG payment in one instance will recoup that loss later on a stay which costs less than the DRG reimbursement. This probably works to a great degree, because most hospitals treat a significant number of Medicare patients. However, the leveling effect for a hospital which files only a handful of Medicaid claims in a year may only be appreciable over a span of time more appropriate to geology than to the health care industry. If a small rural hospital treats a Medicaid patient who has an extraordinarily long and/or expensive stay, under the no-outlier policy they may only receive a fraction of their incurred costs. Moreover, the hospital may be unlikely to treat enough low cost Medicaid clients to make up the difference within a meaningful time span.

Clearly, for these low-volume providers an even more critical issue will be the case mix of Medicaid clients in the base year, particularly while the three-year re-basing system persists. If the base year case mix consists of low cost claims or claims paid relative to the case intensity, the hospital will be penalized with a low SDA until the next re-basing, regardless of its case mix in the interim years. Annual re-basing would help alleviate some of the inequity for low-volume hospitals, and the $1,200 minimum SDA ameliorates the potential negative consequences of a weak case mix in the base year. Nonetheless, it would seem that a more statistically justifiable approach to setting SDAs for providers under some minimum annual volume could be devised, such as an SDA based on longer term trends of those facilities. The THA has supported the creation of some sort of adjustment for low volume and rural providers.[16]

Hospitals which serve large numbers of Medicaid recipients are not immune from being penalized by the PPS methodology. Those which serve large indigent populations, in particular those which perform a large number of deliveries, may end up with an SDA which is skewed downward because normal deliveries are relatively low cost hospitalizations. When those hospitals provide delivery (or other) services at a nominal (below cost) billed charge, the Relative Weight for the DRG for all providers is skewed downward, since these high-volume, low-cost providers shrink the numerator of the Relative Weight calculation.[17] Some adjustment for this latter tendency is indicated, if only to prevent the unintentional penalization of other providers. There is also something fundamentally troubling about a system which penalizes a specific provider for serving a large indigent population. Disproportionate share reimbursement of providers who serve large numbers of low income patients can and has compensated to some extent for the downward skew in SDAs of these hospitals. The disproportionate share program is still very new (disbursements to hospitals were made for the first time in 1987). Whether it will provide adequate compensation will depend on the level of funding for the program and the flexibility of federally imposed definitions of eligible hospitals in future years. A discussion of disproportionate share reimbursement is included in Chapter Nine.

Base Year Data: Impact of Retrospective System's Interim Rates

Under the current PPS, SDAs and Relative Weights are generated from data on claims paid on 1985 HCFA cost reports. In 1985, claims paid to hospitals were factored by what was referred to as the "interim rate". This rate was, for most hospitals, based on data from 1983 cost reports. The interim rate was simply a ratio of claims dollars actually paid to a facility in 1983 to the number of dollars of costs it reported. As such, the rate was intended to reflect the proportion of costs reported which were allowable under Medicaid. In this way the state hoped to limit overpayments to hospitals which it would have then had to recover at final settlement (typically 3 years later) of the cost report. To illustrate, a hospital which in 1983 received payment for 80% of the costs it reported would in 1985 have been paid 80% of all claims submitted, subject to final settlement in 1987 or 1988.

Because of the interim rate, some hospitals can legitimately complain that in 1987 they are being reimbursed according to 1983 data. A hospital with a low interim rate from 1983 but which actually reported a higher percentage of allowable costs in 1985 would have a lower SDA calculated than that to which it was truly entitled, because actual claims paid in 1985 were based on the 1983 rate, and SDAs are based on claims paid, not reported costs. Final settlement of 1985 cost reports is now under way, and hospitals may use the appeals process to adjust SDAs to reflect actual allowable claims for 1985. The possibility also exists that a hospital's SDA could be reduced after such an appeal, if enough reported costs are disallowed.[18]

<u>Relative Weights for Low-Incidence DRGs</u>

Under the current methodology, DRGs for which there were fewer than ten Medicaid incidences in base year 1985 are assigned the Medicare RW for that DRG.

For the base year, there were 26 such DRGs. THA analysts compared the remaining 446 Texas Medicaid RWs with the corresponding Medicare RWs and found that the Texas weights were 25-30% higher than those used by Medicare (the SDA's used by Medicare are much higher than those for Medicaid, though, so typical Medicare reimbursement is higher). The association proposes that TDHS should increase the 26 Medicare RWs by a weighted mean average of 25-30% to put them in proper proportion to the data base.[19]

Rural Hospitals

It is clear that many of the most serious inequities arising from the current PPS methodology are those which affect smaller, typically rural hospitals simply because their Medicaid volumes are too low to generate realistic cost profiles. In general, the rural hospitals of Texas are more concerned with the impact of Medicare than Medicaid, because they do serve relatively few Medicaid patients, whereas Medicare admissions make up 43% of total rural admissions, as compared to 29% for Texas hospitals in general.[20] While the troubles besetting rural Texas hospitals may not be inflicted by Medicaid, the demise of those hospitals will certainly aggravate the problem of access to care for indigents which already exists. Of the 57 Texas hospitals which closed between 1981 and 1986, 41 had 50 beds or less, accounting for 72% of total closures, though hospitals of that size make up only 30% of the total hospital population.[21] In 1987 alone, 27 hospitals in the 50-bed or less category closed.[22] When taken in consideration along with the problems of access to physician care in rural areas discussed in Chapter Seven, a threat to the quality of health care in rural Texas becomes apparent. While improving inpatient hospitalization reimbursement under Medicaid for rural hospitals will certainly not correct the problem by itself, it makes little sense for the state to sustain a policy which may actually contribute to the problem.

Problems with DRGs: Children's Hospitals

Because the DRG system of classifications was developed for the Medicare population of the aged, blind and disabled, it was not designed to encompass all areas of hospital services. The THA has recommended that specialty hospitals for children, cancer patients, or for rehabilitation, and distinct hospital sub-units which serve these populations, should be exempt from the Medicaid PPS until the DRG system is expanded to reflect accurately the complexity of services provided to these special populations.[23]

Special attention has been directed to the situation of children's hospitals. The current set of DRG classifications contains only six classifications for newborns, including only three distinct classifications for premature infants.[24] It is widely recognized that neonatal care of premature infants is some of the costliest hospital care and entails many extraordinarily long stays. The importance of adapting the system is indicated by the large percentage of Medicaid claims generated by patients who are children; in 1985 40% of Texas inpatient care Medicaid claims were for children, and more than half of those claims were for newborns.[25]

The National Association for Children's Hospitals and Associated Institutions (NACHRI) has developed a package of Children's DRGs which are being considered for adoption for Medicare by HCFA. TDHS has studied reimbursement of neonatal cases by Medicaid and has concluded that use of Medicare DRGs results in inequitable reimbursement for high-intensity neonatal care.[26] Software for the new "CDRGs" became available in February of 1988, but is presently being modified to make it compatible with Texas systems. TDHS plans to analyze the potential fiscal impact of the new classifications by applying them to the population of cases in the aforementioned study to see how providers would have been reimbursed under CDRGs. Analysts will assess the degree to which the CDRGs are superior in grouping cases with like costs, and will make recommendations regarding adoption of the system accordingly.[27] THA supports TDHS' interest and efforts, and has recommended implementation of the NACHRI CDRGs.[28]

Even if the NACHRI CDRG system is approved and implemented by TDHS, children's hospitals will still be faced with an enormous uncompensated care bill resulting from the 30-day spell of illness limitation. A recent study conducted by the Wayne State University School of Medicine found that the average length of hospitalization for infants weighing 1500 grams (3.3 lbs.) or less at birth was longer than 30 days for surviving infants. For the smallest babies (500 grams), the average length of stay for survivors was over 95 days, and for the 1000 gram infants the ALOS for survivors was about 65 days.[29]

The impact of these long stays is predictable. The Children's Hospital Association of Texas analyzed Medicaid billings for inpatient hospitalization of children from September 1986 through September 1987.

Total billed charges came to $47,211,158 (for 5928 children), but reimbursement was only $20,972,273, or an average of 44.4%.[30] Children's hospitals also typically are recipients of many transfer patients from general hospitals; thus many patients have exhausted some portion of their 30-day coverage before they come through the door. The children's hospitals point out that Medicare currently exempts children's hospitals from the DRG system, and suggest that this is indication of a consensus at the federal level that the DRG system is inappropriate for Children's hospitals.

Conclusions

There are two kinds of issues entailed in the cases outlined above; equity of reimbursement and adequacy of reimbursement. Equity issues can and should be addressed even in an atmosphere in which only budget-neutral changes can be implemented. However, unless the public sector is prepared to take on the burden of being sole provider of publicly funded hospital care, steps must be taken to insure that providers are also reimbursed at an adequate level to cover costs. Texas cannot expect hospitals to continue indefinitely to provide services for which they receive inadequate reimbursement, no matter how equitably distributed those reimbursements may be. While the position that hospitals should not profit from Medicaid patients is justifiable, hospitals should reasonably expect reimbursement to cover variable costs.

Notes

1. National Heritage Insurance Company, letters to Medicaid providers with attached "Summary: Texas-based DRG Payment System," May 21, 1986.

2. Ibid., pp. 1-9.

3. Ibid, p. 3.

4. Texas Hospital Association, "Technical Advisory Group-Report Number 1: Projected Losses of Texas Medicaid PPS," 1986, p.3.

5. Interview with Rick Peters, Director Inpatient Reimbursement Division, Economic Analysis Division, Texas Department of Human Services, Austin, October 6, 1987.

6. Texas Hospital Association, "Memorandum: Update-Texas Medicaid Prospective Payment System," August 14, 1987, p. 2.

7. Interview with Rick Peters, Director of Inpatient Reimbursement Division, Economic Analysis Division, Texas Department of Human Services, Austin, October 6, 1987.

8. Texas Register, "Proposed Rules," October 7, 1986, p. 4211.

9. Charles Bailey, King Hillier and Dick Kreiter, Texas Hospital Association TAG, "Memorandum Regarding Appeal Rules-Medicaid Prospective System," October 2, 1987.

10. Interview with Rick Peters, Director of Inpatient Reimbursement Division, Economic Analysis Division, Texas Department of Human Services, Austin, October 6, 1987; Rick Peters, letter to Medicaid providers regarding SDA methodology and attached sheet, "Definitions and Calculations Used in Attachment A," dated September 23, 1987.

11. Burnham B. Jones, Senior Vice President, Finance,Texas Hospital Association, "Memorandum: Texas Medicaid PPS Report 1," April 22, 1987, p. 2.

12. Telephone interview with Rick Peters, Director of Inpatient Reimbursement Division, Economic Analysis Division, Texas Department of Human Services, Austin, November 30, 1987.

13. Texas Hospital Association, Technical Advisory Group, "Report Number 3, Texas Medicaid PPS: Status Report of All Activities," October 13, 1986, p. 7.

14. Ibid, p. 6.

15. Ibid., p. 7.

16. Burnham B. Jones, Senior Vice President, Finance,Texas Hospital Association, "Memorandum: Texas Medicaid PPS Report 1," April 22, 1987, p. 3.

17. Texas Hospital Association, "Technical Advisory Group-Report Number 1: Projected Losses of Texas Medicaid PPS," 1986, p.4.

18. Interview with Rick Peters, Director of Inpatient Reimbursement Division, Economic Analysis Division, Texas Department of Human Services, Austin, October 6, 1987.

19. Texas Hospital Association, Technical Advisory Group, "Report Number 3, Texas Medicaid PPS: Status Report of All Activities," October 13, 1986, p. 6.

20. Donna B. Jones, "Rural Hospitals, Changing with the Times," Texas Medicine, vol. 84 (February 1988), p.58.

21. Ibid.

22. Ron J. Anderson, M.D., "The Flip Side of Health Care Expenditures in Texas," Texas Medicine, vol. 84 (February 1988), p.7.

23. Ibid., p. 8.

24. National Heritage Insurance Company, "Texas-based Diagnosis Group Payment System, Revised April 1, 1987 (Revision II)," Austin, April 1987.

25. Gail Bellamy, Stephen Svadlenak, Richard Peters and Donald R. Kelley, "Medicaid DRG System Being Improved for Texas Children," Texas Hospitals, Vol. 43 no. 1, June 1987, p. 14.

26. Ibid.

27. Telephone interviews with Gail Bellamy, Health Policy Analyst, Division of Future Policy Alternatives, Texas Department of Human Services, Austin, December 2, 1987, and May 24, 1988.

28. Texas Hospital Association, "Testimony of the THA: TDHS Public Hearing, Texas Medicaid PPS," December 3, 1986. (Draft.)

29. Department of Pediatrics, Wayne State University School of Medicine, "Average Days in Hospital for Different Birthweight Groups (survivors and non-survivors)," Detroit, n.d. (Photocopied handout.)

30. George Farr, President and Chief Executive Officer, Children's Medical Center of Dallas, Testimony before Select Committee on Medicaid and Family Services, Austin, February 11, 1988, p.5.(Written copy of testimony presented.)

Chapter Six
Long Term Care:
Reimbursement and Eligibility Issues

Although a good deal of the current attention to Medicaid expansion plans has been focused on the under-served working poor, it is also important to examine the status of services to the aged under Medicaid. In 1986 aged Medicaid recipients made up 20.4% of the total eligible population in Texas, and accounted for 24.3% of recipients. Over 40% of all payments for medical services under Medicaid were attributable to these same recipients. Approximately 62% of Medicaid spending for the aged went to long-term care facilities: skilled nursing facilities (SNFs) and intermediate care facilities (ICFs). These and other statistics are displayed in Table 6.1 in order to describe the dimensions of Texas' Medicaid nursing home population.

As the figures in Table 6.1 indicate, services to the aged account for a substantial portion of total Medicaid spending in Texas. Nursing home care for the aged represented 25% of all payments for medical services under Medicaid in Texas.[1]

Because Texas' investment in long-term care of the elderly under Medicaid is so large, a comprehensive plan for expansion of Medicaid should consider changes both in eligibility of the aged and in reimbursement of long term care facilities. This consideration is indicated not only for purposes of evaluation of the cost-effectiveness of the current program, but also because the success of a broad-based expansion plan will depend on support from the community of

Table 6.1
Long Term Care and the Aged Under Medicaid
(Texas, FY 1986)

	Aged	Aged as % of Texas Total	Texas Total
# Recipients Over Age 65	213,305	24.3%	878,985
Total Pymts. for Medical Services	$656,996,954	40.3%	1,628,389,115
# Recipients in Nursing Homes	57,828	90.4%	63,983
Payments for Nursing Home Care	$409,749,767	88.9%	$460,531,576

* Nursing home figures reflect total number of recipients for the year;include SNF and ICF; exclude ICF-MR.

Source: TDHS, Form HCFA-2082, "Statistical Report on Medical Care:
Eligibles, Recipients, Payments and Services," for fiscal year ending September 30, 1986.

---

health care providers, in which the long-term care industry is a significant force. This chapter will describe changes which have been recommended by the long-term care industry and by various independent studies of the long term care situation in Texas. Discussions of these proposals are prefaced by descriptions of the current eligibility and reimbursement systems.

Eligibility of the Aged

As was noted in an earlier chapter, all Supplemental Security Income (SSI) recipients are eligible for Medicaid in all states. Beyond that population, states may at their discretion extend coverage to persons residing in Medicaid approved nursing homes who meet SSI eligibility criteria (age 65 or older, blind or disabled), and whose income exceeds the SSI Federal Benefit Rate (FBR) of $340 (1987) but is less than or equal to three times the FBR, or $1020 in 1987. These persons must also meet resource eligibility requirements; that is, their assets other than income are also considered. This nursing home population is the only SSI-related population which may spend down to Medicaid eligibility in Texas. This population of Medicaid recipients is referred to as SSI-related MAO (for Medical Assistance Only). Persons found eligible for Medicaid under either category may also submit to Medicaid any unpaid medical bills incurred in the three months prior to application if they met all the eligibility criteria during that three-month period. Several categories also exist which guarantee continued eligibility to institutionalized recipients who were originally enrolled under more liberal eligibility guidelines.[2]

Texas has established a special income limit which for the year 1987 is $658.65 for the SSI-MAO population. Of the fifty states, 19 have Medically Needy/Spend down programs, 22 states use the maximum allowable limit of $1020, and nine states (including Texas) use a special income limit which is lower than the maximum. Of those nine, only one state, Delaware, adopted a more restrictive rate than Texas in 1986.[3] It should be noted that states have considerable latitude in determining resource requirements, and can thereby engineer the size of the SSI-related Medicaid population to a greater degree than if income level alone were discretionary.

Application of Medicaid to Nursing Home Care

An understanding of the mechanics of the payment of nursing home bills for Medicaid recipients is helpful in understanding the potential costs of changing the eligibility cap. As noted, Texans over age 65 must have countable income of less than $658.65 and must also meet strict resource tests in order to receive Medicaid. When a Medicaid eligible person enters a nursing home, all of his countable income except for a monthly personal needs allowance (PNA) of $30 is applied to his bill. Medicaid pays only for the difference between the Medicaid approved monthly rate for the facility and the patient's income (less PNA). Persons who are receiving SSI payments (monthly countable income less than $340) when they first enter a nursing home "lose" the SSI benefit after the first month of care; however, they are immediately reassigned to the MAO program, so no interruption of service results from this nominal change in status.[4]

Changing the SSI-Related MAO Income Limit

It has already been noted that only one state uses a more conservative SSI-MAO income limit than Texas. The 70th Texas Legislature, in the house version of the 1988-89 Appropriations Bill, considered lowering the income limit to $609 a month in FY 1988 and FY $509 a month in 1989. The Texas Department of Human Services (TDHS) estimated that 8,780 nursing home residents would have lost eligibility under the proposed eligibility cuts. There is no way of knowing what might have become of these persons had the reductions been pursued. Certainly some of them would have had to leave the facilities where they were receiving care, and ultimately the legislature opted to maintain the current eligibility limit along with a very small cost of living allowance to reflect the federal increase in the SSI FBR.[5]

The 70th Legislature received recommendations from a number of groups regarding the problems of long-term care in Texas. Among the groups which addressed the eligibility cap issue were the Texas Long-Term Care Coordinating Council for the Elderly, the Committee on Health and Human Resources of the Texas Senate, the Texas Silver-haired Legislature, and the State Board of Insurance Long-term Care Advisory Group. All of these groups recommended raising the cap.[6]

How Much Will It Cost?

Putting a price tag on such eligibility increases is difficult. It is far simpler for TDHS to project the impact of decreases in eligibility because the population affected is already completely defined. In order to accurately project the cost of an increase, the number of persons who meet the income guidelines must be known. Somehow an estimate of that portion of those income-eligible persons which would also meet resource standards must be made. This is of course a good deal more difficult. Once the dimensions of the newly eligible population have been estimated, projections of utilization must be made; for example, how many persons who have been receiving care in the home from family members chose to move into nursing homes when they become eligible for Medicaid. To what degree will currently institutionalized self-pay clients take advantage of new eligibility?

The Texas Long-Term Care Coordinating Council for the Elderly (LTCCCE) reported to the 70th legislature projections provided to the committee by TDHS analysts which indicated that the cost of increasing the eligibility cap to the maximum allowable limit for the 1988-89 biennium would have been $19.4 million for the state, based on a state's share of 43.09% for 1988 and 40.96% for 1989. The LTCCCE projections were based on the extension of services to an additional 9,175 persons.[7]

Analysts at TDHS note that the LTCCCE figures assume that the income eligibility cap would be raised for in-home care waivered clients as well as for the institutionalized aged population. Unofficial in-house projections from TDHS reflect similar utilization patterns, but are based on the smaller population of about 7,400 resulting from the exclusion of those in-home clients. The state's share for this smaller estimate would be about $16.6 million. However, based on extrapolations from the income and resource distribution of the current Medicaid eligible population, TDHS officials have expressed concern that these earlier estimates of cost may in fact be too low.[8]

Either estimate may sound improbably low for a 35% increase in the eligibility ceiling of a program for which over $531 million has been appropriated for FY 1988. Proponents of raising the eligibility limit point out that the population which would benefit from a more generous income limit is an "inexpensive" one in that only the gap between their income (which is more than $658.65 but less than $1020) and the federal maximum of $1020 would be picked up by Medicaid, and that only 40-43% of that difference would be borne by Texas.

OBRA 1987 included provisions which will eliminate the distinction between SNF and ICF facilities by 1990 by making the standards for all homes the same. The legislation established minimum standards which will be applied to all homes for staffing by registered and licensed practical nurses, and for training levels and competency evaluations for nurse aides. Homes with more than 120 beds will be required to employ at least one full-time social worker. Special federal funds will be available during 1988 and 1989 to help offset new costs attributable to nurse aide training and evaluation.[9] TDHS has not projected what these improved standards will cost the state in higher reimbursement, but increased costs will certainly be significant.

Personal Needs Allowance

The personal needs allowance (PNA) for nursing home residents receiving Medicaid had remained the same at $25 since 1974.[10] OBRA 1987 raised the PNA to $30, effective January 1, 1988.[11] Nursing home care typically does not include the price of prescription medicines and Medicaid in Texas will pay for no more than 3 prescriptions per month. Although pharmacists are highly cooperative in helping to stretch Medicaid recipients' prescription allowances, many elderly persons require so many prescriptions that they must spend some or all of their personal needs allowance on drugs.

Even those who do not have to dip into this allowance for prescription medicines find that $30 will not go very far towards providing personal amenities which may make life in a nursing home more pleasant. For those without significant family support the $30 budget must provide any "extras" such as books, magazines, newspapers, personal grooming items, stationary, etc. While the size of the PNA is a peripheral issue, it is one which is frequently mentioned in conjunction with proposed changes in the way Medicaid works for Texas nursing home residents. TDHS projects that the cost to Texas in 1988 of paying the state's 43% share of the $5 increase in the PNA will be $1,335,790.[12] Any increases in the PNA which a state makes unilaterally (not mandated by federal law) would be paid for entirely from state funds. If the PNA for the 1986 utilization level of 79,141 aged, blind or disabled SSI and SSI-MAO nursing home recipients[13] (residents of ICF-MRs are already eligible to retain up to $75 of personal earnings[14]) were raised to $50 in 1986, the cost to Texas for footing the additional $20 per recipient would be almost $19 million if every recipient was eligible for the PNA.

Reimbursement of Nursing Homes under Medicaid

Reimbursement of nursing homes by Texas' Medicaid program is moderately complex, but a basic understanding of its workings is worthwhile inasmuch as it makes possible an evaluation of the nursing home industry's criticisms of the current system.

Each Medicaid qualified nursing home must submit an annual cost report to TDHS. TDHS auditors eliminate entirely certain reported costs deemed "unallowable" and place caps on certain others. Remaining costs are allocated to four categories: (1)administration costs, (2)facility costs, (3)dietary costs and (4)patient care costs. A statewide median cost for each category is then calculated; however, the method of calculation of that cost differs between categories.

The formula for determining the statewide rate is simplest for dietary and patient care costs. The allocated cost for the given category (dietary or patient care) in the base year is adjusted for inflation and then grouped with the allocated cost for that same category from every other Medicaid qualified nursing home. The median of all these values, adjusted to yield a daily cost, serves as the dietary or patient care component of the rate. Separate calculations of patient care costs are done for ICFs and SNFs in order to generate different rates for the two.

The derivation of the facility cost rate is identical to that of the dietary and patient care categories, except that each facility with an occupancy rate below 85% has an occupancy adjustment applied to its allocated cost for the category before the median value for all homes is calculated. The rationale for this adjustment is to eliminate the counting of empty beds in the calculations. The formula for reaching an individual homes' facility cost is given below (this example is for a home with occupancy below 85%).

{(percent occupancy)/(85)} x {facility costs}

Depreciation costs are allocated to facility costs. Homes which have changed hands after 1984 may only depreciate against a facility value based on the pre-1985 facility cost increased by one-half of the urban inflation rate.

In the administration cost category, the same occupancy adjustment used for facility costs is applied to each nursing home's administration costs. When all the resulting occupancy-adjusted administration costs are grouped together, TDHS eliminates the top 15% from consideration before calculating the median. This adjustment is intended to reduce the possibility of homes benefitting from incurring greater administrative expenses, and to limit the extent to which large nursing home chains can pass on their central office expenses to individual homes (and thus to the state).

The resulting set of rates is very simple; there is one daily rate for SNFs, one daily rate for ICFs, and a single supplemental rate, SNL1 (service need level 1) for SNF patients who are determined to require extraordinary care. These rates are calculated by adding the median dietary and patient care costs to the adjusted medians calculated for administration and facility costs. Rates are based on cost reports generated two years previous to the current date, so that 1988 rates are based on 1986 cost reports. For 1988 these rates are $47.17, $34.64 and $7.59 respectively.[15]

Issues in Reimbursement Methodology

The Texas Health Care Association (THCA) has raised a number of questions regarding the current methodology in rate-setting for nursing homes. The Association commissioned a study of the methodology in 1986, the results of which were reported to the 70th Texas legislature. A summary of those results identified several areas of contention.

Allowable Costs

The current reimbursement methodology requires that depreciation of facilities be based on a 40-year lifetime with a ten percent salvage value, despite the fact that federal regulations require only a 30-year lifetime.[16]

THCA argues that costs are disallowed which are well within generally accepted accounting principles. The cost of self-insuring for worker's compensation is not treated as an allowable cost, though purchased worker's compensation insurance can be treated as a cost. Expenses entailed in fund-raising are not allowable as costs, but any funds raised must be deducted from the amount of costs which Medicaid will reimburse. Also disallowed are costs such as filing fees, director's fees and costs of filing federal income taxes, though these costs are unavoidable for incorporated facilities.

Adjustments to Costs

The THCA study takes issue with the adjustments to administration and facility costs, pointing out that the effective rate at which administration costs are reimbursed is the 42.5 percentile. It is important to recognize that it is the median and not the mean value of the cost array which goes into the rate-setting formula, so that the skewing effect of extreme cost outliers is already quite limited; thus the 15% cut is something of a double hit. One effect of this adjustment is that older facilities which have a good deal of equity (which is not reflected in the rates) and relatively low occupancy may register costs just above the median in the first array. Occupancy adjustment often pulls them below the median, with downward rate revision resulting for all facilities.

Also notable in the facilities cost is the limitation (implemented under TEFRA) of allowable depreciation and interest costs for homes sold after

1984. This provision was a laudable attempt to prevent the artificial inflation of rates through multiple resales of facilities. Unfortunately, the methodology is too rigid to reflect legitimate increases in fair market value.

It is clear that the objective of the adjustments to facility and administration costs is to create an incentive for nursing homes to minimize those costs and to thereby concentrate spending on services which directly enhance the quality of patient care. However, the THCA study makes the compelling point that administrative and facility costs (facility costs include depreciation, interest, maintenance and repairs, leases, etc.) are basically fixed or semi-fixed costs. Nursing homes which need to cut down on costs in response to reimbursement rates because those rates do not cover incurred costs can be expected to make cuts in variable cost areas; namely, in dietary and patient service expenditures. Furthermore, reductions in expenditures in these areas today will translate to lower reimbursement rates two years down the line, which might then result in further cutbacks in patient service spending.

<u>Adequacy of Cost Coverage</u>

THCA's study reported that in 1985 over $44 million in costs were disallowed under the current system. Illustrative of the impact of the magnitude of the disallowances is the THCA study's finding that when the books of the 926 nursing homes which made up the 1985 rate-setting population were used to calculate profit or loss, 404 homes showed a loss before taxes. The size of the loss was substantial enough that the average home lost $0.74 per patient day before taxes.

However, when TDHS cost disallowances are taken, the average home shows a net income of $0.81 per patient day.[17]

Another notable finding of the study was that reimbursement rates for administration and facility costs projected for 1987 using the 1985 cost report data are actually lower than the average audited allowable costs for 1985, although there is certainly no reason to think that the cost of care has decreased since 1985.[18]

Is the THCA's claim that Medicaid reimbursement does not cover the cost of care valid? The report to the 70th legislature by the State Board of Insurance provides figures that suggest that at minimum there exists a large disparity between private pay and Medicaid reimbursement. In 1985, the average cost of care in a Texas nursing homes was $21,900 for a private home, $22,403 for a Veterans Administration facility, and $20,746 for ICF-MRs. In that same year, payment for the average Medicaid ICF client was $11,107, and payment for the average Medicaid SNF patient was $15,133.[19]

It seems unlikely that the intensity of care provided to the clients of these different payors is inherently different enough to justify this difference in reimbursement. It seems more likely that in nursing home care, as in other areas of health care, cost-shifting to private pay patients is subsidizing the public sector payor client. In a sense our current policy amounts to taxation of the paying clients, or of the long-term care industry. The question of whether this is the way Texas really wants to fund long-term care for the poor elderly is worthy of consideration.

Case Mix Intensity

THCA claims that one of the causes of increased costs to nursing homes in recent years is the implementation of the Diagnostic Rate Group (DRG) prospective reimbursement system under Medicare[20] (presumably Medicaid DRG use has the same effect). Reimbursement for inpatient hospitalization beyond the number of days calculated as average length of stay (ALOS) for a given condition is extremely limited. As a result, there is a strong incentive to discharge patients earlier than may be indicated in an individual case. One result of this is that patients are, on the average, coming to nursing homes in a more frail medical condition and are requiring more a more intensive (and thus more costly) level of service.

As noted above, the only recognition by Medicaid of such variations in intensity of services rendered by nursing homes is in the SNL1 supplement. In an attempt to redress this weakness in the reimbursement methodology, TDHS has undertaken a demonstration project which will test a more complex case mix system. The experiment will begin in July of 1988 and will compare nursing home clients in five counties using the experimental system with those in four control counties using the current methodology.

Under the trial system, patients will be assigned to one of 13 categories according to the intensity of services which they require. Case mix categories are sometimes given the generic appellation of "RUGs" (for resource utilization groups) after the prototype New York State case mix system. However, Texas' index for assignment to a case mix group is called the Texas Index for Level of Effort (TILE), so both acronyms may be encountered in discussions of the Texas system. Prospective per diem rates will be calculated for each of the 13 groups. These groups will only be applied to the patient care portion of the cost calculation; the other three categories will be calculated according to the current methodology. The case mix of a facility will be reevaluated twice a year.

Although this system clearly does not address every complaint with the methodology outlined above, the experimental case mix system will offer reimbursement which reflects directly the unique costs of patient care incurred by individual facilities in the experimental group.[21] However, it is reported that the state plans for the system to be revenue neutral. If this is the case, the system will address equity issues only, and will have little impact on adequacy of reimbursement.

Indications for Change

Why should Texans be concerned about nursing home reimbursement under Medicaid? First, as noted above, nursing home care accounts for a considerable portion of the Medicaid budget, so taxpayers should be concerned about the fair and efficient use of Medicaid funds. Also, Texas will need more nursing home beds in the future. Currently there is no shortage of nursing home beds in Texas as there is in many other states; in fact, in 1987 the average occupancy rate for Texas nursing homes was 82% compared to national averages of 90-95%.[22] In 1986 the Texas Department of Health reported 104,066 nursing home beds available.[23] However, it is projected that by the year 2000 Texas will need between 152 thousand[24] and 197 thousand[25] total nursing home beds. The is some evidence that the crunch will first be felt in the form of a shortage of beds available for the most resource intensive patients. In Dallas, for example, it has been claimed that over one half of SNF level IV nursing home beds have been closed over the last four years, and are being replaced by less intensive (and hence more profitable) beds.[26] This trend underscores the need for adoption of some sort of case mix program like the aforementioned TILE system. It is also true, however, that the changes in staffing requirements instituted by OBRA 1987 will have the effect of raising all Texas homes up to the SNF level of services, so this trend may soon be irrelevant.

The "Boren Amendment" of the Omnibus Budget Reconciliation Act of 1981 mandated that states reimburse nursing homes at rates which are reasonable and adequate to meet costs of care in conformity with all applicable state and federal standards. Beyond this legal obligation, another justification for public concern over Medicaid reimbursement of nursing homes is that if we expect entrepreneurs to invest in long-term care facilities to meet this demand for beds which we anticipate, we must be prepared to provide a level of reimbursement for public-payor clients which will cover the costs of care at an acceptable level of quality. Failing that, we can expect the result generally associated with inadequate price ceilings; that is, demand will exceed supply. And, in such a situation, we would be surprised to find high quality patient care. If Texas wants to avoid getting into the nursing home business, adequate reimbursement is essential.

Recommendations

The cost benefits of expanding Medicaid eligibility for nursing home residents are not as obvious as the benefits of certain other expansions because cost-shifting to local payors of last resort is not as explicit. Who bears the cost when an elderly person whose income exceeds the eligibility cap by some small amount is denied Medicaid? What happens if there are no family members around to either pay the gap between the person's income and the cost of private pay nursing, or to take care of the elderly person at home? The answers tend to differ according to local conditions. However, the argument that the taxpayers of Texas ultimately benefit from a bigger return on their federal tax dollars applies to all areas of the Medicaid program. Justification for increasing the personal needs allowance to $50 is not to be found in cost analysis; rather, the change is indicated on the grounds that it is a relatively inexpensive move which will create a more humane and dignified situation for the Medicaid recipients in nursing homes.

As noted previously, there is a sound market-based justification for making changes in nursing home reimbursement. Implementation of a statewide case mix system will result in more "reasonable and adequate" reflection of true costs; likewise, the accounting principles applied to reported costs must be adapted to reflect the real operating costs of nursing homes. Placing caps on administrative costs and salaries may be necessary and justifiable. However, sound accounting principles would seem to mandate the allowance of corporate fees and self-insurance. The disallowance of fund-raising expenses is particularly baffling in that it essentially creates a disincentive for facilities to raise funds, despite the fact that donations would directly reduce the state's expenditures on the facility.

Changes in eligibility and reimbursement for nursing home care must be included in a Medicaid expansion plan for several reasons. First, the support of the long-term care industry will be essential if Medicaid expansion is to be funded and implemented. Also, it is essential that the nursing home industry be able to operate in a favorable climate, because the problems of financing long-term care for all Texans will only become more profound with the passing years. Medicaid is only a part of the long term care picture, but it is sensible to utilize the resources available under Medicaid optimally until a better system is devised. Finally, of course it is not enough that facilities be able to cover costs and that an adequate supply of Medicaid beds exists. Rates must also be adequate to support a high quality of care, and standards should be monitored and enforced to ensure that high quality.

Notes

1. Texas Department of Human Services, Form HCFA-2082, "Statistical Report on Medical Care: Eligibles, Recipients, Payments and Services," for fiscal year ending September 30, 1986.

2. Texas Department of Human Services, "Medicaid Eligibility in Texas (Title XIX)," January 1, 1987. (photocopied guidelines prepared for Rep. Jake Pickle)

3. Letter to Texas Health Care Association from Barry Fredrickson, Assistant Commissioner of Client Services Branch, Texas Department of Human Services, April 9, 1987.

4. TDHS, "Medicaid Eligibility in Texas (Title XIX)," January 1, 1987. (Prepared for U.S. Rep. Jake Pickle)

5. Senate Bill 1, General Appropriations Bill for Fiscal Years 1988 and 1989, art. II, sec. 29(10) and art. II, sec. 39(30).

6. Texas State Board of Insurance, The Long Term Care Dilemma: What Can Be Done About It?" January 1987, pp. 45-51. (Report to the 70th Texas Legislature)

7. Texas Long-Term Care Coordinating Council for the Elderly, "Recommendations to the 70th Legislature," December 1986, p. 4.

8. Telephone interview with David Cook, Director of Budgeting, Services to Aged and Disabled, Texas Department of Human Services, November 20 and 24, 1987.

9. Omnibus Budget Reconciliation Act of 1987, P.L. 100-203, sections 4211-4218.

10. Interview with Dorothy Crawford, Executive Assistant for Government Relations, Texas Health Care Association, Austin, October 1, 1987.

11. Omnibus Budget Reconciliation Act of 1987, P.L. 100-203, section 9119.

12. Texas Department of Human Services, "Federal Legislation Briefing: Select Committee on Medicaid and Family Services," Austin (December 4, 1987), Part IV, p.6. (Photocopied for distribution to Select Committee on Medicaid and Family Services.)

13. Texas Department of Human Services, Form HCFA-2082, "Statistical Report on Medical Care: Eligibles, Recipients, Payments and Services," for fiscal year ending September 30, 1986.

14. TDHS, "Medicaid Eligibility in Texas (Title XIX)," January 1, 1987. (Prepared for U.S. Rep. Jake Pickle)

15. Texas Department of Human Services, Agenda Item no. 4, Meeting of Texas Board of Human Services, December 17, 1987, p.2.

16. Texas Health Care Association, Executive Summary of study of Nursing Home Reimbursement Methodology, March 1987. (copy of material provided to 70th Texas legislature)

17. Ibid.

18. Ibid.

19. Texas State Board of Insurance, The Long Term Care Dilemma: What Can Be Done About It?" January 1987, p. 27. (Report to the 70th Texas Legislature)

20. Jerome Chapman, Executive Director of Texas Health Care Association, testimony before Texas House of Representative Budget and Oversight of Human Services Committee, February 25, 1987.

21. Texas Department of Human Services,"Nursing Home Case Mix Demonstration Project," October 21, 1987, (draft) as cited in briefing paper prepared by Linda Logan.

22. Jerome Chapman, Executive Director, Texas Health Care Association,"From Old Folks Homes to the Medical Model," 1987.(adapted from speech to first annual Gerontological Conference of the University of Texas Health Science Center at Houston)

23. Texas State Board of Insurance, The Long Term Care Dilemma: What Can Be Done About It?" January 1987, p. 19. (Report to the 70th Texas Legislature)

24. Texas State Board of Insurance, The Long Term Care Dilemma: What Can Be Done About It?" January 1987, p. 22. (Report to the 70th Texas Legislature)

25. Healthcare Financial Management Association, Long-Term Care: Challenges and Opportunities (Oak Brook, Illinois, 1985), p.42.

26. Ron J. Anderson, M.D., "The Flip Side of Health Care Expenditures in Texas," Texas Medicine, volume 84 (February 1988), p. 7.

Chapter Seven

Reimbursement of Physician Providers

In fiscal year 1986, Texas physicians were reimbursed $152,598,272 by Medicaid for services provided to 59,748 recipients.[1] Reimbursement of physicians involves questions of equity and adequacy with respect to the provider, and access to and quality of care for the recipient. The methodology now in use is described in this chapter, along with issues concerning that system and the implications for Medicaid recipients.

<u>Reimbursement Methodology</u>

The methodology used for the reimbursement of physicians by Texas Medicaid is borrowed from the Medicare program. Like reimbursement for inpatient hospitalization, the program is currently contracted out to the National Heritage Insurance Company (NHIC), which uses the Blue Cross-Blue Shield reimbursement data base generated for Medicare. This methodology is also used to reimburse providers such as ambulance services, medical laboratories and medical supply companies. The amount of payment is determined by comparison of each charge with two standards, with the amount paid being the lesser of either of the two standards or the actual billed charge itself. The two standards for comparison are the Customary Charge and the Prevailing Charge.

To calculate the customary charge, NHIC constructs a profile for each individual M.D. which details the amounts which he or she billed during a twelve-month period for various procedure codes. All charges filed during that period for the same procedure are arrayed (some adjustments are made for extreme outliers), and the lowest charge which is high enough to include the median value of the array is designated as that provider's customary charge for that procedure. Individual billings can thus be compared to the physician's historical charges for treating the same condition.

A doctor must have billed for a given procedure at least three times in the year to establish a customary charge. If a physician has not established a customary charge, if he changes specialties, or if he relocates to a new locality (as defined by the methodology), his payment will be based on the 50th percentile of the prevailing charge profile.

Prevailing charge profiles are created to make possible comparison of the billed charges of doctors in the same locality who are practicing the same medical specialty. Localities are defined by NHIC. Counties with populations of 50,000 or more are designated as locality. There are 30 such county localities. Counties with less than that number of residents are grouped into one of three regional localities.

At least four physicians practicing the same specialty in the same locality must all have generated customary charge profiles in order to develop a prevailing profile for that locality and specialty. If there are not enough specialists in a county or even a regional locality to generate a profile, doctors are compared at the next higher aggregate level; that is, regionally or even statewide.

Prevailing profiles array the customary charges of the physicians involved, weighting those charges to reflect how often that provider performed that procedure during the year. The prevailing charge is considered to be the 75th percentile of that array. As mentioned above, the 50th percentile of the array is used to reimburse physicians who have not established customary charges.

In theory, customary charge profiles are to be recalculated annually. However, as is the case in most provider reimbursement programs, the data being used at any given time will typically be at least one and one half to two years old. NHIC anticipates recalculating the customary profiles in the spring of 1988; the data which will be used to generate the new profiles will be charges from January 1986 through March 1987.[2] Since the prevailing charge profiles are generated from those customary charges, it is clear that the former will of necessity lag even a bit further behind.

A 1972 amendment to the Social Security Act, P.L. 92-603, provided that when the prevailing charge profiles are updated, the resulting increase cannot exceed the levels for the year 1973 by more than "the extent justified by economic changes as reflected in appropriate economic index data." The effective ceiling for Medicare and Medicaid created by this law is referred to as the economic index limitation (EIL).

The economic index used by the two programs is calculated annually and is fairly complex. Weighted values for increases over the previous year in housing costs, transportation costs, pharmaceutical prices, hourly earnings in several white-collar professions, malpractice insurance premiums, and other miscellaneous expenses derived from the Consumer Price Index (CPI) are combined and multiplied by 40%. This weighting is based on the assumption that 40% of a doctor's income goes to expenses, with the remaining 60% going to net income. An index which reflects the annual increase in average weekly earnings of production and non-supervisory workers and the output per man hour of employed non-farm workers is multiplied by 60% to allow for an increase in net income.[3]

Profile Methodology Issues

The significance of the use of this index is suggested by the fact that it is consistently significantly lower than the CPI; a TMA report found that between 1975 and 1980 it ranged from a low of 49% to a high of 68% of the CPI. Physicians have suggested that while use of the EIL has certainly reduced the immediate payout for Medicaid and Medicare, it may have also contributed to increased cost-shifting to private patients and a heavier burden on Medicare recipients whose doctors do not take assignment. It has also been pointed out, however, that this cost-shifting could only take place if physicians were charging less than the market will bear, or if demand for medical services were highly price inelastic.

Physicians may bill their Medicare patients for amounts above the reimbursement level, a practice referred to as "balanced billing". As such, adequacy of reimbursement is not as pressing an issue from the physician's point of view (clearly it may be an issue to the Medicare recipient who must pay the difference) in Medicare as it is in Medicaid, where the reimbursement amount must be accepted as payment in full. This fact calls into question the use of the same reimbursement schedule for the two programs.

TMA also holds that rural providers carry a special burden. The cost differential between urban and rural practices which existed when the EIL legislation passed has virtually disappeared in the intervening years; however, the practical effect of the EIL is to make it impossible for rural providers to ever catch up to the urban reimbursement standard.[4] Another unintended effect of the ceiling is that it creates a disincentive for physicians to locate in rural localities if they anticipate serving significant numbers of either Medicaid or Medicare patients, since the prevailing profiles in urban areas are so much more favorable for reimbursement.

Other Reimbursement Issues: Texas Medical Association

The Texas Medical Association (TMA) has expressed support for expansion of eligibility and services under Texas Medicaid.[5] Recent recommendations by the TMA Council on socioeconomics to the membership included several items related to Medicaid. TMA is advocating repeal of the 10% across-the-board reduction in reimbursement which was placed in effect in 1985 for all Medicaid hospitals and physicians in response to state budget woes. Also recommended was the establishment, at the request of the TDHS Deputy Commissioner for Health Care Services, of a special advisory committee to meet with him to address issues relating to the Medicaid program. The Council also commended TDHS for its expressed concern about the adequacy of reimbursement for obstetrical (OB) care, and recommended that TMA assist the Department in identification of a more equitable reimbursement structure for such care.[6]

The Medicaid Obstetrics Problem

The underlying concern with the adequacy of OB reimbursement is that insufficient reimbursement may result in a lack of physicians willing and available to deliver Medicaid babies. Access to OB care by Medicaid recipients is a growing problem nationwide. In December of 1987, five California Medicaid recipients filed a class action suit demanding that the state improve access of indigent citizens to medical care. One of the plaintiffs in the suit is a Medicaid recipient who, after contacting 40 doctors, was unable to find one who would provide obstetrical services and accept Medicaid as payment. Business Week estimates that reimbursement for OB care by Medicaid in California is "typically" about 40% of the amount which Blue Cross-Blue Shield would pay for the same services. The deputy director of California's Health Services Department has stated that the state is considering funding improved rates for OB care by reducing reimbursement for other physician services, an approach which certainly will not appeal to physicians, and which may only aggravate problems of adequacy in other service areas.[7]

While inadequate reimbursement may be a national problem in Medicaid obstetrics, the problem goes beyond obstetrics in Texas. A recent study compared reimbursement in Medicaid programs in the 50 states plus the District of Columbia. Texas was given good marks for nursing home and inpatient hospitalization reimbursement, but physician reimbursement was singled out as being exceptionally low. Physician payments in Texas of $441 for an appendectomy and $518 for complete obstetrical care (adjusted for varying wage costs from state to state) are significantly lower than the national median payments of $714 and $1,201 for those procedures.[8]

While the threat of lawsuits and the costs of liability insurance create problems across all medical specialties, the liability problems of obstetricians present special problems for Medicaid. There are several reasons why this is the case. First, poor women are less likely to have received adequate prenatal care, which places them at higher risk of having a difficult delivery and which increases the risk that their infants will have medical problems. In addition, indigent mothers also tend to be younger. To illustrate, Parkland Memorial Hospital in Dallas reports that the majority of patients served by the MIHIA program there are between the ages of 13 and 20.[9] Their young age itself associates these women with a higher risk of "poor pregnancy outcomes" such as low birth weight. It is therefore not surprising that indigent mothers are said to be statistically the most likely patients to sue a physician.[10]

In Texas, TMA has collected data on the attitudes of physicians towards Medicaid, and their responses to those perceived problems. A study commissioned by the association and conducted in August of 1986 found that the career-long incidence of lawsuits filed against Texas OB-Gyn specialists is 125 per 100 doctors; that is, the average OB had been sued at least once in his career. Only the surgical specialties report a higher incidence of suits, and the average rate for all specialties is 79 per 100. Twenty-five percent of OB-Gyns who have been sued at some point in their careers have been sued by indigent patients who are not under the physician's continuing care, although those same doctors reported that indigent patients made up only 10% of their overall patient load. When asked to what degree either experience with suits filed by indigent patients or fear of the same had caused them to limit their service to indigent patients, 35% of OB-Gyns replied that they had limited services "a great deal", 14% replied "some" and another 5% said they limited services "just a little".

It would be inaccurate to attribute this conservative behavior on the part of doctors simply to fear of incurring lawsuits. Whatever a physician's personal perception of risk and his willingness to assume the same may be, the reality is that the cost of malpractice insurance for those doctors who deliver babies is significantly higher than for those who do not. The above-mentioned TMA study found that not only 37% of Family and General Practitioners but also 14% of OB-Gyns reported having eliminated obstetrics completely from their practices as a way to save money on insurance.[11]

This is yet another area in which the impact of the problem is particularly severe in rural Texas. According to a survey conducted by Randy Fritz in 1985, only 15% of OB-Gyns in Texas practice outside the large metropolitan areas. Because of this, small towns and rural areas are especially dependent on General and Family Practitioners. In this survey 65% of Family physicians responding said that they no longer delivered babies, an even greater proportion than was found in the TMA study. Further, the author found that the greatest proportion of that 65% were those who practice in rural areas.[12] The results of these studies confirm that a serious deficit in medical services in rural areas is developing; also, the lack of access to OB care in rural areas is no doubt adding to the burden of large public providers in the metropolitan areas.

Figures collected by the Texas Medical Liability Trust in 1987 illustrate rather starkly the financial disincentives to providing OB services. Rates quoted were for a five-county area including Houston. For a family practitioner performing no surgery to purchase $1-2 million in coverage, the premium was $4,957. The same practitioner performing major surgery without deliveries would pay $15,605, and if he delivered babies the rate would be $20,657. For the same coverage, an obstetrician paid $47,428.[13] It is easy to see that a family doctor would have to generate a good deal of income from deliveries or from surgery in order to be able to justify the cost of offering these services to his patients. In a rural or small town setting often a caseload sufficient to cover the insurance costs will not exist.

Some more subtle effects of these high insurance expenses on Texas' Medicaid program are suggested by a other data collected in the 1986 TMA study. When doctors were asked how they planned to handle future increases in liability insurance premiums, 69% said they would pass the increases through to their non-Medicaid, non-Medicare patients.[14] Since insurance costs represent such a large expense, it is easy to see how the kind of disparity in reimbursement which was illustrated in the California case will come into being if the Medicaid methodology is not flexible enough to accommodate those costs. Regardless of where one feels the seat of responsibility for the increase in liability insurance costs lies, physicians must pay those premiums until such a time as a solution is found. As long as Medicaid reimbursement rates do not reflect these true costs, a disincentive will exist for physician participation in the program.

It is also worth noting that concerns about liability may result in an upward creep in costs to all patients, including Medicaid patients. In practicing what has been referred to as "defensive medicine" (also characterized at times as "bad Medicine"), doctors increase the levels of testing, consultations and even hospitalizations they recommend, beyond what they may feel is strictly necessary to diagnose and treat a patient. This is done in order to establish for any future jury or judge that the doctor has gone to every prudent length possible in the provision of care. Respondents in TMA's survey estimated that about 13% of their patients' bills could be attributed to such costs.[15]

Very little research or print has been devoted to determining what the impact of existing Medicaid reimbursement is on quality of care provided by physicians to Medicaid patients. We have seen that access to physician care (outside of public hospitals and clinics) is often limited, but what happens when a recipient does find a private practitioner willing to accept Medicaid as payment?

One of the original selling points for passage of Title XIX was the hope that it would bring provision of health care for the poor into the mainstream, so that a person with a Medicaid card would be as welcome in a doctor's office as the person covered by Blue Cross-Blue Shield. Conventional wisdom indicates that this is certainly not the reality in Texas. Instead of the mainstreamed approach desired by the program's creators, we find that certain physicians are referred to as "Medicaid Docs". And, though some of these practitioners are no doubt motivated by a desire to serve the low-income population, other physicians tend to associate such practices with "bad medicine".

It seems that here, as with nursing home reimbursement, adequacy of reimbursement is needed not just to guarantee access to care, but also to assure that Medicaid recipients will have access to the same quality of care as the rest of the population. A system of physician reimbursement which is adequate to cover true costs, is no more inconvenient for the facility than private third-party reimbursement, and which incorporates strict utilization review procedures (focused on both quality and cost) should be implemented if the Medicaid approach is to be retained. Otherwise, Texas and the country as a whole could just as well establish a second-tier public health system for the indigent in which the government would be free to keep a close eye on quality of care and cost efficiency.

In summary, although the liability "crisis" transcends the bounds of the Medicaid population, some of the most immediate negative effects of the problem are being felt in the area of indigent health care in general. Attention to the problem of OB disenrollment is indicated, as a deficit in access to care will undermine the effectiveness not only of the MIHIA program, but also that of any future implementation of the OBRA 1986 and the 1988 options for children and pregnant women. Some sort of indemnification or government supported risk pool for Medicaid providers is one possible approach to the problem; another would be simply to assure that reimbursement rates reflect true costs of liability insurance. In either case, stricter review of quality of care would be essential.

Notes

1. Texas Department of Human Services, Form HCFA-2082, "Statistical Report on Medical Care: Eligibles, Recipients, Payments and Services," for FY 1986 (Austin, January 1987), pp. 6, 34.

2. Telephone interview with Doreen Cardenas, Provider Enrollment, National Heritage Insurance Company, Austin, March 22, 1988.

3. Larry L. Tonn, Texas Department of Human Services, "Calculation of the Economic Index Factor," (Photocopied report prepared for informational use), August 20, 1981, pp. 1-2.

4. Ad Hoc Committee on Physician Reimbursement, Texas Medical Association, "Report to the Texas Medical Association Executive Board," April 5, 1981, pp. 72-74.

5. David Vanderpool, M.D., President, Texas Medical Association, Cover letter to information packet for Select Committee on Medicaid and Family Services, February 11, 1988.

6. Texas Medical Association, "Report of Reference Committee on Socioeconomics," November 1987, pp. 7-8.

7. Susan B. Garland and Gail DeGeorge, "A Welfare Mother's Battle to Clean Up the Medicaid Mess," Business Week, no. 3031 (December 21, 1987), p. 42.

8. Karen Erdman and Sidney M. Wolfe, M.D., Poor Health Care for Poor Americans (Washington, D.C.: Public Citizen Health Research Group, 1988), p. 181.

9. Ron J. Anderson, President and Chief Executive Officer, Parkland Memorial Hospital (Dallas, Texas), Testimony before Lieutenant Governor's Select Committee on Medicaid and Family Services, Texas Legislature, Austin, February 17, 1988, p. 5.(Written copy of testimony presented.)

10. Texas Medical Association, "Documenting the Crisis: A Survey of Texas' Primary Care Physicians," (Enclosure in packet of information provided to Select Committee on Medicaid and Family Services), Austin,

February 11, 1988.

11. Texas Medical Association, "Documenting the Crisis: A Survey of Texas' Primary Care Physicians," (Enclosure in packet of information provided to Select Committee on Medicaid and Family Services), Austin, February 11, 1988.

12. Randy Fritz, "A Physician Survey of Texas' Liability Crisis: Impacts on Indigent Patient Care," (Summary reproduced by Texas Medical Association of a study done at LBJ School of Public Affairs, University of Texas at Austin, 1985).

13. "Professional Liability Premiums (TMLT) 10/87: Maximum Rates after 4 Years Claims," (Figures provided by Texas Medical Association to Dr. Donald Kelley, deputy Commissioner for Health Care Services, Texas Department of Human Services, October 26, 1987).

14. Texas Medical Association, "Documenting the Crisis: A Survey of Texas' Primary Care Physicians," (Enclosure in packet of information provided to Select Committee on Medicaid and Family Services), Austin, February 11, 1988.

15. Ibid.

Chapter Eight
The Vendor Drug Program

The Vendor Drug Program is responsible for reimbursing providers of prescription drugs under Medicaid in Texas. The reimbursement methodology for prescriptions is somewhat simpler than are those used by the other provider programs. The formula used to calculate the amount a pharmacy will receive for a given prescription is:

$$\frac{\text{(Statewide Dispensing Exp.)} + \text{(Acquisition Cost of Drug)}}{0.945}$$

If, however, the price which a given pharmacy most frequently charges the general public for the same drug (the Usual and Customary Price) is less than this calculated amount, the provider will be reimbursed at that lower rate. Freestanding pharmacies which offer free delivery of prescriptions to Medicaid recipients receive a flat ten cent per prescription add-on to the calculated rate. The manner in which each term in the above equation is calculated is explained below.

Statewide Dispensing Expense

Any pharmacy which dispenses an average of at least 200 Medicaid prescriptions per month in a base year (defined as the 12-month period ending three months before the end of that pharmacy's fiscal year) must file an annual cost report with TDHS. This cost report is a 14-page document which collects both demographic data and data on allowable expenses of the pharmacy. From these data TDHS calculates a per-prescription mean dispensing cost for the pharmacy. The median value of the array of individual mean dispensing costs of all the reporting pharmacies is the

Statewide Dispensing Expense which is used to reimburse every pharmacy. This value is recalculated annually, and remains in effect for the full calendar year. In 1987, the value used was $3.26.[1]

Every cost report is desk audited by the Vendor Drug Program. The Program also maintains a staff of regional pharmacist auditors who perform on-site audits of pharmacies.

Estimated Acquisition Cost of a Drug

Pharmacies may purchase drugs either directly from a manufacturer or through a wholesaler. The Estimated Acquisition Cost (EAC) for a drug purchased from its manufacturer is the actual amount paid for the drug, subject to verification by TDHS. If, however, the drug is purchased from a wholesaler, the EAC is considered to be the lesser of either (1) the published Red Book Average Wholesale Price (AWP) minus 10.49% or (2) the wholesalers own cost plus 12%.[2] Excepted from this policy are controlled ("scheduled") prescription pharmaceuticals. Because they can rarely be purchased at less than Red Book price, the EAC for these controlled substances is the unadjusted AWP.[3]

Opportunity for Profit

The sum of the EAC and the state wide dispensing fee is divided by 0.945, resulting in a 5.5% profit directly related to the selling price of the drug.[4] The incorporation of a profit portion related to the selling price (as opposed to a flat per-prescription enhancement) by Texas was disputed by HCFA. HCFA's position held that the profit percentage constituted a mark-up which was inconsistent with Medicaid policy of paying costs only.[5] Texas' methodology has been vindicated by a subsequent change in HCFA policy which now explicitly allows the opportunity for profit. However, prior to the rule change HCFA did disallow some claims for reimbursement on this basis, and final settlement of TDHS' appeal of the disallowance is still pending.[6]

Non-Legend Drugs

Non-legend drugs are drugs which can be dispensed without a prescription. Doctors prescribe such drugs, even though they can be obtained over the counter, so that their costs may be covered by a third-party payor such as Medicaid. Insulin is an example of a non-legend drug which is often prescribed. The Vendor Drug Program will not pay for some non-legend drugs such as diet pills and certain types of vitamins.

Reimbursement for covered non-legend drugs is the lower of the provider's usual and customary charge or the EAC of the drug plus 50%; no dispensing fee is included.[7]

Texas Maximum Allowable Cost

The Vendor Drug Program has implemented the Texas Maximum Allowable Cost (TMAC) program to promote the use of generic ("multi-source") drugs. Texas' program is one of the most aggressive in the country, as it includes virtually all generic drugs available.[8] TDHS estimates that TMAC saved the program $11.6 million in 1987.[9]

Multi-source drugs which are therapeutically equivalent are grouped together and the median of their wholesale estimated acquisition costs is the maximum allowable EAC to be used in the reimbursement formula. Thus, if a pharmacy chooses to provide a more costly form of the generic drug prescribed, it will take a loss on the transaction. Providers who supply forms of the generic with acquisition costs lower than the TMAC cap do not reap a profit, but are reimbursed at the lower price which they actually paid.[10]

TDHS adjusts the TMAC limit in some circumstances. For example, there are instances in which the supply of a generic drug at or below the TMAC limit may not be adequate to meet the demand for the drug. In such a case, the TMAC cap would be raised. Physicians may also override the generic program by specifying on the prescription form that a particular brand name is necessary.[11]

Hospital Pharmacies

Under current regulations, hospital pharmacies are reimbursed according to the same basic standards as freestanding pharmacies, except that the flat statewide dispensing expense is reduced by half before calculation of the reimbursement amount.[12] Proposed changes to the reimbursement methodology would extend the 50% reduction in the dispensing expense also to dispensing physicians.[13] Hospital pharmacies are not required to file cost reports.[14] Hospitals have traditionally had access to prices for drugs purchased direct from the manufacturer which are significantly lower than those available to many pharmacies. Other implications of differential pricing by drug manufacturers are discussed in the section below.

Issues in Vendor Drug Reimbursement:

The Pharmacies

How good a deal does the Vendor Drug Program offer to Texas pharmacies? First, it should be noted that Vendor Drugs is the only reimbursement program in which the threat of provider disenrollment is not a recurring theme. Nonetheless, there are aspects of the methodology which are seen as problematic by pharmacies. Also, an understanding of the VDP must begin with recognition that the program has to accommodate the interests not only of pharmacies and pharmacists, but also those of physicians and of the drug manufacturers. The direction and focus of cost containment efforts in the Texas VDP has followed the line of least resistance; that is, the bulk of controls have been aimed at pharmacies, which are the least powerful of the three involved interest groups. The following paragraphs deal with some of the practical effects on pharmacies resulting from the methodology, and some of the Texas Pharmaceutical Association's (TPA) stands on the methodology and the VDP generally.

Under current regulations, physicians may prescribe up to a six-month supply of most drugs. Though Texas Medicaid recipients are limited to three paid prescriptions per month, the six-month supply rule stretches the prescription allowance quite a bit further than would be possible if doctors could only prescribe up to a 30-day supply, as is the case in most states. As a result, the cost attached to the average individual Medicaid prescription claim in Texas is much higher than the national average. The flat statewide dispensing fee given to pharmacies by the VDP is also one of the highest in the nation, but because this flat fee is applied to a greater total selling price per prescription, the effective gross margin is actually very low, and is said to be among the lowest in the nation.[15]

Although the VDP does concentrate on cost containment, higher-cost drugs are still used extensively. Medicaid's cost-intensive elderly recipients are much more likely to be taking various prescription drugs on a daily and ongoing basis than are their younger counterparts in the program. Moreover, doctors naturally tend to prescribe the products which they consider to be "state of the art". One example of such a drug is Tagamet, which is commonly prescribed for ulcers and other gastrointestinal problems and which is also taken routinely by many older persons. Since Tagamet is still under patent, no generic substitutes are available, and the drug is one of the most commonly prescribed for Medicaid recipients in Texas.

One rationale for including an opportunity for profit in the reimbursement formula is that this enhancement compensates to some degree for the costs of maintaining an inventory of these expensive name-brand drugs. It is estimated that 65-70% of participating pharmacies are small independent businesses which cannot benefit from the economies of scale available to the large chain pharmacies.[16] For these providers, inventory maintenance can represent a substantial expense. The TPA would like to see the opportunity for profit increased to at least seven percent.[17]

The state could exercise the option to contract with low-bidding providers to supply Medicaid prescriptions. Such an approach would need somehow to take into account the location of such providers. One reason such a high percentage of services is provided by small independent pharmacies is that the large chains do not locate in the areas where poor people (i.e., Medicaid recipients) live. Provision of Medicaid prescriptions by the large pharmacies which can submit lower bids for but which recipients cannot easily get to would not represent an improvement in the delivery system.

As was noted in the explanation of VDP reimbursement methodology, if the usual and customary price charged by a pharmacy is less than the amount which would result from use of the formula, that usual and customary price is used to reimburse the pharmacy. Any discount which would have applied to the Medicaid recipient had he been purchasing the prescription himself (prices to third-party payors are not considered) must be considered usual and customary.[18] One practical implication of this policy is that by offering a senior citizens' discount, a pharmacy automatically lowers its usual and customary price profile for Medicaid customers age 65 and older. While this has not been a major issue for pharmacies, it does create an questionable disincentive for offering seniors substantial discounts.

<u>Containing Manufacturers' Prices</u>

Both the TMAC program and the methodology for calculation of the EAC are highly effective cost-containment measures which derive savings entirely through controlling the profit margin of pharmacies, rather than through any direct controls on the prices charged by drug manufacturers. A 1987 study by TDHS estimated that costs of dispensing drugs (pharmacy costs) account for 20% of the Vendor Drug Program's total reimbursement costs, with the actual cost of the pharmaceutical making up the remaining 80%. The study concluded that if further cost reductions are to be achieved, the logical target will be reductions in the prices charged by manufacturers.[19]

Whatever the apparent logic may be, practical means with which Texas might address the manufacturers' costs of pharmaceutical may be limited. Texas has, in fact, discussed the adoption of a Manufacturers Rebate program.[20] In such a program a drug manufacturer would rebate to the state the difference between the price it charged to pharmacies for products ultimately supplied to Medicaid recipients and some previously agreed upon price (such as the price charged to non-profit institutions) to be charged Texas Medicaid. In theory, a rebate program would allow the state to take advantage of whatever clout it may have as a potential quantity buyer without actually having to take over the purchasing and distribution of pharmaceutical. In its 1987 report on the feasibility of implementing a rebate program, TDHS estimated that Texas Medicaid accounts for only about 10% of the prescription drug business in the state, and concluded that this percentage is not large enough to eliminate the possibility that manufacturers might choose non-participation in Texas Medicaid over compliance with the rebate program.[21]

While a thorough discussion of the problem of controlling prescription drug costs is beyond the scope of this report, several points can be made. First, it has been well established that the prices of prescription drugs have been increasing at a rate far greater even than that of general health care costs, which have themselves accounted for the greatest increases in the Consumer Price Index over the last decade. It is also clear that drug manufacturers do engage in differential pricing, often offering prices to major institutional buyers which are far lower (even below cost in some cases) than those available to pharmacies of any size. In fact, TDHS cited as a major objection to the rebate program its concern that the implementation of a rebate might threaten Texas' access to low bids for state institutions' drug purchases.[22] While saving on institutional purchases at the expense of the VDP sounds like false economy, it may well be true that the savings Texas would achieve through a rebate program might not offset potential losses in institutional pricing. At present it would seem that direct reductions in manufacturers' drug prices under Medicaid are most likely to be accomplished at the federal level, where much stronger incentives for manufacturer cooperation could be realized.

Utilization Control: A Medicaid Formulary?

The Texas Pharmaceutical Association went on record in 1987 urging TDHS to "consider establishment of a state formulary system limiting the number of drugs covered (by the VDP), especially generics."[23] The VDP at present uses the Texas Drug Code Index (TDCI) as its formulary. The TDCI includes virtually all FDA-approved legend and non-legend drugs, excluding anti-obesity drugs, adult vitamins, immunizing agents, some kinds of children's vitamins and multiple-ingredient anti-anemia products.[24] What TPA is advocating would be a much more restrictive formulary aimed at containing costs by limiting the use of more expensive drugs.

Drug formularies are used by most third-party health care payors to list which drugs they will cover. The degree to which formularies are used for cost control (beyond that derived from the exclusion of products of questionable therapeutic value) varies extensively. The use of a very strict formulary could be anticipated to draw some opposition from the pharmaceutical industry since their profits could be affected. Physicians' associations may also express concern regarding the institution of a strict formulary on the grounds that it would interfere with the physician's ability to offer the best possible care to a patient.

<u>AIDS and Medicaid: AZT</u>

In December of 1987, the Texas Board of Human Services approved the addition of azidothymidine (AZT) to the TDCI. Prior to the effective date of January 1, 1988, the costs of AZT used by Medicaid patients with AIDS or AIDS-related complex (ARC) were not covered by the VDP. Texas was one of the last states to add AZT to its Medicaid formulary after FDA approval of the drug in March of 1987 and the announcement in the following month by HCFA that states could cover AZT under Medicaid.

Concern about the cost of the addition was the reason for the delay. The average per-patient cost of AZT has been estimated to be about $8,500 a year; however, Burroughs-Wellcome, the manufacturer of AZT (marketed as Retrovir), reduced the wholesale price of the drug by 20% in December of 1987, so the average cost may drop for 1988.[25] The overall price tag for AZT is expected still to be quite high. Although TDHS has made no official projections of the cost, unofficial estimates have ranged from $500,000 to $1,000,000 per year.[26] The Vendor Drug Program had already anticipated a deficit of $15-18 million for the 1988-89 biennium prior to the addition of AZT,[27] and since the 70th legislature appropriated no additional funds to support the addition of AZT to the

VDP there is understandable concern that cuts in other critical areas of the program will have to be made to fund the deficit.[28]

Under the newly adopted policy, coverage of AZT would be subject to certification by a licensed physician that the Medicaid recipient has AIDS or ARC, and that any patient with a history of chemical dependency is under therapy for that condition. The Texas Department of Health has also received a federal grant funding AZT for low-income AIDS patients who are not eligible for Medicaid. The VDP plans to use the purchase and distribution system established by TDH under the AZT grant program, which will allow Medicaid to take advantage of the low price and discounted dispensing fee already negotiated by TDH.[29]

It is also worth noting that the use of AZT carries along with it new costs other than just the cost of the drug itself. The very success of the drug therapy will result in higher lifetime costs for AIDS patients simply because they live longer. It has also been suggested that the harsh side effects associated with AZT may result in a need for more intensive outpatient care or even additional hospitalizations.[30] A new drug, inhalation pentamidine, is expected to gain wide use in the fight against AIDS at a projected cost of several thousand dollars per patient per year, and at least sixty other new drugs are being tested for use in AIDS treatment.[31] Clearly the VDP will be one of the programs most strongly affected by the extraordinary costs associated with AIDS.

Medicaid Expansion and the VDP

The extension of Medicaid to a larger population of poor Texans would not seem to directly create or to aggravate any issues with the providers associated with the Vendor Drug Program. Overall, as the program expands the greatest concern of the pharmacy providers will probably continue to be the historical tendency to place the entire burden of cost control on the pharmacy rather than the drug manufacturer or the physician. Despite the fact that the latter two factions wield relatively greater power than the pharmacies, a move towards the use of a stricter formulary seems inevitable. As previously noted, unless the state becomes a direct contractor with the pharmaceutical companies, it will be difficult to control the manufacturers' costs at the state level, though effective action could be taken at the Federal level. Since the Vendor Drug Program has probably extracted the maximum tolerable savings from the pharmacies themselves, any future cost cutting will have to be derived from some other source.

Notes

1. Title 40, Social Services and Assistance, Part I, Texas Department of Human Services; Chapter 35, Pharmacy Services, subchapter F, Reimbursement, section 35.9001(a)(2).

2. Texas Department of Human Services, Feasibility Study- Drug Manufacturers Rebate Program: Why a Manufacturer's Rebate? (Austin, February 1987), p.4.

3. Telephone interview with Pat Gladden, Director of Policy and Audit, Vendor Drug Program, Texas Department of Human Services, Austin, February 19, 1988.

4. Title 40, Social Services and Assistance, Part I, Texas Department of Human Services; Chapter 35, Pharmacy Services, subchapter F, Reimbursement, section 35.9001(d).

5. Interview with Ken Kirk, Phd., Associate Dean, School of Pharmacy, University of Texas at Austin, Austin, January 14, 1988.

6. Telephone interview with Pat Gladden, Director of Policy and Audit, Vendor Drug Program, Texas Department of Human Services, Austin, February 19, 1988.

7. Title 40, Social Services and Assistance, Part I, Texas Department of Human Services; Chapter 35, Pharmacy Services, subchapter F, Reimbursement, section 35.601(3).

8. Interview with Ken Kirk, Phd., Associate Dean, School of Pharmacy, University of Texas at Austin, Austin, January 14, 1988.

9. Texas Department of Human Services, Feasibility Study- Drug Manufacturers Rebate Program: Why a Manufacturer's Rebate? (Austin, February 1987), p.5.

10. Title 40, Social Services and Assistance, Part I, Texas Department of Human Services; Chapter 35, Pharmacy Services, subchapter F, Reimbursement, section 35.604(c).

11. Title 40, Social Services and Assistance, Part I, Texas Department of Human Services; Chapter 35, Pharmacy Services, subchapter F, Reimbursement, section 35.606(a).

12. Ibid., section 35.9001(d)(3).

13. Texas Department of Human Services, "Reimbursement Methodology for the Pharmacy Dispensing Fee," Austin, January 1988. (Draft of proposed methodology.)

14. Ibid., section 35.9001 (b)(1)(A).

15. Interview with Ken Kirk, Phd., Associate Dean, School of Pharmacy, University of Texas at Austin, Austin, January 14, 1988.

16. Interview with Ken Kirk, Phd., Associate Dean, School of Pharmacy, University of Texas at Austin, Austin, January 14, 1988.

17. Texas Pharmaceutical Association, "Pharmacy Management: Third Party Programs," item 58, adopted 1987.(Official adopted stands of the TPA)

18. Title 40, Social Services and Assistance, Part I, Texas Department of Human Services; Chapter 35, Pharmacy Services, subchapter F, Reimbursement, section 35.604.

19. Texas Department of Human Services, Feasibility Study- Drug Manufacturers Rebate Program: Why a Manufacturer's Rebate? (Austin, February 1987), p.9.

20. General Appropriations Act, Section 63, art. 2, 69th Texas Legislature (September 1, 1985).

21. Ibid., pp. 9, 12.

22. Ibid., p. 8.

23. Texas Pharmaceutical Association, "Pharmacy Management: Third Party Programs," item 56, number 4, adopted 1987.(Official adopted stands of the TPA)

24. Texas Department of Human Services, Legislative Appropriations Request FY 1988-89, July 7, 1986, p. 2:324.

25. Ron J. Anderson, M.D., "The Flip Side of Health Care Expenditures in Texas," Texas Medicine, vol. 84 (February 1988), p.8.

26. Richard Thomas Conlon, The Medical Cost of AIDS, (Professional Report, Lyndon B. Johnson School of Public Affairs, University of Texas at Austin, December 1987), p. 76.

27. Telephone interview with Patricia Gladden, Director of Policy and Audit, Vendor Drug Program, Texas Department of Human Services, Austin, February, 1988.

28. Marlin W. Johnston, Commissioner, Texas Department of Human Services, Recommendation to Texas Board of Human Services, "AZT Coverage in the Vendor Drug Program," agenda item no. 8(December 1, 1987), pp. 1-2.

29. Ibid., p. 2.

30. Richard Thomas Conlon, The Medical Cost of AIDS, (Professional Report, Lyndon B. Johnson School of Public Affairs, University of Texas at Austin, December 1987), pp. 37, 39.

31. Ron J. Anderson, President and Chief Executive Officer, Parkland Memorial Hospital (Dallas, Texas), Testimony before Lieutenant Governor's Select Committee on Medicaid and Family Services, Texas Legislature, Austin, February 17, 1988, p. 13.(Written copy of testimony presented.)

Chapter Nine
Local Funding Options

Across-the-Board Local Participation

States have the option under Title XIX of using local funding as part of the non-federal share of their Medicaid budget. Some limitations apply to this option; state funds must account for at least 40% of the total amount which is put up to be matched by federal funds. It is stipulated that if a state elects to use local financial participation, a lack of funds from a local source may not result in a diminution of services of any kind to that particular jurisdiction.[1]

A number of states use local funding as part of their state's share. Table 9.1, below, provides a list of those states and a brief description of the funding formulas used.

Table 9.1
Local Funding Formulas for Medicaid Vendor Payments
As of March 31, 1986

Colorado	20 largest counties pay 2% of state's share for all new ICF admissions.
Florida	Counties pay lesser of 35% of cost or $55 per month for each nursing home resident; 35% of cost for inpatient hospital days over 12 and less than 46.
Iowa	Counties match federal funds for ICF-MRs.
Minnesota	Counties pay 10% of the state's share.
Montana	Counties pay 18% of eligibility workers' costs.
Nebraska	Counties pay 4.67% of total expenditures.

New Hampshire	County pays approx. 28% of nursing home costs (excludes state facilities); also some institutional costs for aged and blind.
New York	Counties pay 50% of non-federal share, except for long-term care for which they pay 28% of non-federal, 20% in 1986.
N. Carolina	Counties pay 15% of non-federal share for all services.
N. Dakota	Counties pay 15% of state share except for ICF-MRs, clinic services, and waivered community and home based services for MR, aged and disabled.
Pennsylvania	Counties pay 10% of state's share for county nursing homes plus administration fee of $3 per invoice.
South Dakota	County pays $60 per month for each ICF-MR resident and local school district for crippled children's hospital.
Utah	County contribution of less than 1% for specific services (eg., mental health).
Wisconsin[2]	Counties which operate nursing homes may apply amount, if any, of operating deficit towards FFP.

Source: U.S. Department of Health and Human Services, Health Care Financing Administration, Analysis of State Program Characteristics, 1986, Table 68, Draft Copy. Updated states noted.

All of the states using some form of local funding collect at the county level. In some states the county participation is limited to a few targeted services such as nursing homes and ICFs, while several states the county is obligated to pay a fixed proportion of the state's share of most Medicaid services.

Texas may wish to consider a system of county contributions to the state Medicaid program as an alternative to finding new state appropriations to allow eligibility expansion. Under the Indigent Health Care and Treatment Act of 1985, county responsibility for indigent health care was clarified. As originally passed, counties which were not entirely served or not served at all by a hospital district or a public hospital were responsible for the provision of health care to the indigent in areas of the county not served by the district or the public hospital.[3] Legislation passed by the 70th legislature released city hospital authorities from responsibility for indigent health care, and made it possible for most city-owned public hospitals (all those in cities with populations under 15,000) to contract with the county to assume responsibility for outpatient services provided to indigent persons.[4] As a result, virtually all counties not completely served by a hospital district now have some responsibility for indigent care.

Since counties have this statutory responsibility to provide health care to the indigent they are logical candidates for consideration as a supplemental funding source for the Medicaid program. A participation formula based on Medicaid utilization such as those used by several of the states listed in Table One might be feasible, particularly since expanded Medicaid eligibility would reduce the size of the population which the county would be obligated to serve without the benefit of matching funds. A county's contribution to the Medicaid fund might be counted towards the 10% of general revenue levy which a county is required to expend on mandatory health care services before becoming eligible to receive state assistance. Another option would be to provide the same type of temporary shelter against a rollback election which the counties were given under the Indigent Health Care and Treatment Act.[5]

Hospital Districts and Indigent Health Care

Should the state contemplate a county contribution system, some parallel mechanism would need to be devised for those counties served by hospital districts, since the hospital district assumes all obligation to provide health care to indigents in such counties. Hospital districts provide a very significant portion of the total amount of health care delivered in Texas; El Paso, San Antonio, Dallas, Ft. Worth, Houston, Amarillo (Randall county is partially served by the Northwest Texas Hospital District), Lubbock, Midland and Corpus Christi are all in counties completely served by these districts. In 1987 there were 77 Texas counties which were completely served by hospital districts.[6]

The Indigent Health Care Act did not define eligibility or responsibility for hospital districts, because the constitutional authority for hospital districts did not specifically empower the legislature to do so. The only new requirement of hospital districts under The Act was that they adopt certain application procedures for indigent patients.[7] Hospital districts were instructed to "provide the health care services required under the Texas Constitution and the statute creating the district."[8] The constitution requires that the districts "assume full responsibility for providing medical and hospital care to needy inhabitants of the county," but no definition of the needy population is provided.[9]

Because the Indigent Health Care Act specifically excluded the hospital districts, a large portion of the state was to a great extent untouched by the legislation. As an initial remedial measure, the 69th legislature passed a proposed constitutional amendment which was approved by the voters in November of 1985. This amendment allows the legislature to create laws determining the services districts must provide and the eligibility requirements they may use, "and any other relevant provisions necessary to regulate the provision of health care to residents."[10] However, to date no implementing legislation has been created.

As it stands, despite the great progress made by the Indigent Health Care Act, there are still 77 Texas counties and portions of 20 others in which responsibility for provision of health care to the poor is basically undefined.[11] In the urban hospital districts in many cases both the eligibility standards and the level of services for the medically indigent are more generous than those required of counties under the law. However, within the group of entities which falls under the constitutional label of "hospital district" there is a great degree of variation in the level of services each provides. Some districts have been created by law but remain inactive and do not levy taxes or provide any services. Other districts levy taxes to support limited services such as nursing homes or emergency medical services. While these low-activity districts are bound by the same vague constitutional obligation as their large urban counterparts, there is no mechanism to guarantee that the obligation is met.

It is expected that legislation clarifying the indigent health care responsibilities of the hospital districts will be passed in future sessions. For some districts compliance with an explicit obligation will require extensive changes, but if the hospital districts can, like the counties, be granted such benefits as state assistance and per patient liability caps, resistance to inclusion under The Act may be limited.

Texas will probably need to take such steps to establish a truly uniform statewide standard for indigent health care before a local contribution to Medicaid will be feasible. It is always a challenge in Texas to try to develop policies which are flexible enough to take into account the vast differences in conditions which exist across the state. As noted above, hospital districts are not a homogeneous group. A very broad range of economic resources exists among the districts. The 70th Texas legislature saw the dissolution of four hospital districts and the creation of eight others. Some hospital districts were created with more limited taxing authority than the 75 cent per hundred dollar valuation limit imposed by the constitution, which may limit their capacity to meet their obligation to provide services to the indigent. Also, a recent opinion of the Texas Attorney General has held that hospital districts are subject to tax rollback election.[12] Legislation defining the indigent health care responsibilities of hospital districts will need to accommodate these differences just as it would the differences in resources between Texas counties.

Such legislation may have the added benefit of hastening either the development or the dissolution of inactive districts, thereby simplifying the jurisdictional situations in counties containing several districts.

If Texas does extend the provisions of the Indigent Health Care Act to the hospital districts, a system of local contributions to Medicaid could be more easily implemented and administered should lawmakers opt to do so. Until hospital districts are brought under the state's indigent health care umbrella, the responsibilities and resources of obligated jurisdictions will be too uneven to allow for an equitable contribution system.

Donated Funds as a Portion of the State's Share

Another funding option, the use of donations as a part of the state's share of the Medicaid program, is currently available under Medicaid regulations. Acceptable sources of a state's share of financial participation are outlined by federal regulation.[13] The regulations allow for both public and private funds to be used as State's share.

Donations from public sources may take several forms: (1) those appropriated directly to a state or local (where applicable) Medicaid agency, (2) those transferred to a state or local Medicaid agency from another public jurisdiction and thus under direct control of the Medicaid agency, or (3) funds certified by the contributing agency as representing expenditures eligible for federal financial participation (under this third option, there need not be an actual transfer of funds to the state Medicaid agency). Contributing public agencies must be able to demonstrate that the funds being used to draw federal match did not originate with the federal government, unless such a use is specifically allowed.[14]

Donations from private sector sources may be added to the state's share only if they are first transferred to the state or local Medicaid agency and are thus under direct administrative control of that agency. Those private funds "[may] not revert to the donor's facility or use unless the donor is a non-profit organization, and the Medicaid agency, of its own volition, decides to use the donor's facility."[15]

History of the Current Regulation

The allowable use of public and private donated funds was restricted to application to personnel training costs until December of 1985.[16] In publishing the revised regulations, HCFA declared its objective to be the removal of "unnecessary requirements in the regulations...that will improve program administration relating to...sources of the state's share of financial participation."[17] Supplementary information provided by HCFA along with the regulations acknowledged that economic pressures on states to find new sources of funding for Medicaid had led to increased interest in the use of donated funds. The restriction of donations to training uses was done "to prevent donations that could be conditional on some benefit to the donor," and thus to avoid any kind of kickback situation.[18] Since subsequent "experience ha[d] shown no abuse of public and private funds through conditional donations or kickbacks,"[19] HCFA concluded that limitation of donations to training alone created the burdensome necessity for states to document that donations and their associated federal-match funds were spent exclusively on training. Furthermore, under the old regulations states which received donations in excess of training costs were unable to apply those extra funds towards other Medicaid expenditures.

Responses to public comments on the regulatory changes were also published in the Federal Register. One comment asked if, under the proposed regulations, for-profit organizations would be prohibited from receiving Medicaid reimbursement if they also had donated funds to the state Medicaid program. The HCFA response simply reiterates the agency's intent without clearly addressing the question, saying,

> section 433.45(b) of the regulations does not prohibit a for-profit facility from participating in Medicaid. It serves only to define what non-state funds may be considered share of financial participation. Our intent is to preclude 'kickback situations' that could result from private donations made by proprietary organizations in return for Medicaid business.[20]

The allowability of donations from for-profit sources which are also Medicaid providers is clearly of importance in assessing the utility of the donated funds approach. Interpretations of this aspect of the regulation are noted in the discussion which follows of several states' donated funds initiatives.

The Regulatory Impact Statement which accompanied publication of these changes in the Federal Register stated,

> We expect little change from current levels of donations to State Medicaid programs as a result of these

> provisions. To the extent that donations increase, the individual state programs will benefit, but we believe that the extent of the incremental increase will not be great enough to benefit affected recipient populations.[21]

Apparently, HCFA failed to anticipate the large scale donation programs which developed in a number of states. This fact seems to account for HCFA's resistance today to implementation of matching of donated funds. Major initiatives by several states and the HCFA response to those plans are described below.

Texas

While Texas is not currently involved in uses of donated funds which involve a great deal of money, one program which is in place has historical significance. The regulatory changes discussed above were to some extent a response to controversy over Texas' early attempts to draw federal match for funds (approximately $175 thousand per quarter) donated by public and private hospitals for the hiring of in-house Medicaid eligibility workers. HCFA disallowed the contributions, holding that instead of being directly matched (50% donated-50% federal match) the contributions should have simply been used to reduce the amount of state funds appropriated for the program and eligible for federal match (50% donated-25% state funds-25% federal match). In other words, HCFA felt that any savings to the state should have been shared with the federal government.

TDHS appealed the disallowance to the grant appeals board of the U.S. Department of Health and Human Services (USDHHS), saying that there was no basis in federal regulation for HCFA's position and that Texas' plan was consistent with HCFA's overall support for alternative funding sources for and increased private sector involvement in human services. The grant appeals board ruled in favor of HCFA.

Subsequent to these rulings, the regulatory changes specifically permitting donations were put into place. Texas appealed the decision of the grant appeals board to Federal District Court, which held that the original decision had no valid basis and therefore directed the grant appeals board to reconsider Texas' case. On the occasion of this second review, the grant appeals board found in favor of TDHS.[22]

As noted, this program does include the donations of for-profit hospitals to be matched. In support of this policy, TDHS held that the payment of eligibility workers (who are state employees) was primarily of benefit to the Medicaid client. As it provided no direct monetary benefits to the hospitals, the program did not create the sort of "kickback situation" which HCFA wished to preclude. Apparently the grant appeals board concurred with this opinion, as they upheld the Texas eligibility workers plan.

West Virginia

West Virginia has suffered in recent years from state Medicaid appropriations so inadequate that between 1980 and 1986 the state carried a backlog of unpaid provider claims which by 1986 approached $50 million.[23] Since HCFA regulations require that most Medicaid bills must be paid by the states within 30 days (certain bills may be paid within 90 days) or the state will be subject to penalty, West Virginia incurred penalties during that period of approximately $250 thousand.[24]

In 1985 West Virginia passed legislation instituting a tax on hospitals which was patterned loosely after that of Florida. The formula for taxation was based on a hospital's percentage of profits factored by its Medicaid payor mix so that, for example, a more profitable hospital which serves relatively few Medicaid patients would pay a higher tax, while unprofitable hospitals with substantial Medicaid populations might not pay at all.

Funds from the taxes collected were deposited in a Medically Indigent Fund of the Health Care Cost Review Authority for the explicit purpose of supplementing state general appropriations to the Medicaid program. This legislation was passed as a temporary measure (to last one year), but in 1986 a modified version of the original legislation, H.B. 2182, extended the levy indefinitely.[25]

Even with the addition to the Medicaid budget of the new tax revenues and their associated federal match, the payment backlog of $50 million persisted in 1986. In the fall of that year, West Virginia Governor Arch A. Moore, Jr. proposed to hospital C.E.O.'s that they make donations to the Medically Indigent Fund with a goal of eliminating the backlog. Since West Virginia receives a generous federal match (about 72.5% in 1987)[26], every dollar donated will be almost tripled. While the proposal had the backing of the state hospital association,[27] some hospital officials reportedly felt at the time that these contributions were not entirely voluntary. It has also been reported that part of the Governor's proposal was to indirectly assure the return of funds to the donating sources by increasing the rate of reimbursement on all hospital charges.[28]

Contributions were received in the amount of $10.4 million. In October the West Virginia Department of Human Services (DHS) filed a revised HCFA-25 along with a cover letter explaining that $10.4 million of the October through December quarter's total was generated by voluntary contributions from hospitals. The HCFA-25 is a report submitted quarterly to HCFA by state Medicaid agencies in which estimates of Medicaid expenditures for the upcoming quarter are provided. Federal matching funds are remitted "up front" to the states based on these estimates.. The HCFA regional office in Philadelphia was consulted about the state's intentions prior to this submission, and HCFA did not express concern.[29] Matching funds for that quarter were provided by HCFA without incident or comment.[30]

Donated funds were not submitted for January-March of 1987. In February of 1987 a letter and a HCFA-25 form reporting more hospital donations were filed for the April-June quarter, but on this occasion an Associate Regional Administrator of the U.S. Department of Health and Human Services (USDHHS) advised DHS that there were indications that the program did not comply with 42 CFR 433.45. The specific manner in which the state failed to comply was not stated, but the letter nonetheless requested that the state discontinue the use of hospital donated funds. In a conversation with a DHS commissioner, the USDHHS administrator expressed concern that the proceeds resulting from the fund donations were primarily being applied to inpatient hospital claims, rather than being used for across-the-board Medicaid expenditures.[31]

In March, the Regional Administrator of USDHHS advised the state that its request for medical assistance award for the April-June quarter would have to be revised because donated funds for that quarter did not qualify as part of the state's share for federal matching funds. The letter also notified the state that official disallowance of the October-December donations was forthcoming. Again, no specific explanation was offered for the funds being considered ineligible. Disallowance notification dated April 2 was received shortly thereafter.[32]

Civil action was filed in U.S. District court by the Commissioner of the West Virginia DHS which resulted in USDHHS being preliminarily enjoined from disallowing the donated funds for the April-June quarter. The decision seems to have been based partly on USDHHS' failure to provide an explanation of the basis of their decision. Also, the disallowance process and the associated appeals process is normally based on disallowance of expenditures already made in a previous quarter. There was apparently no precedent for HCFA's prospective reduction of the state's April-June estimates of available state funds, and thus the proper avenue for appeal of the HCFA action was unclear. The judge also held that the West Virginia donations plan was in keeping with "a fair and reasonable construction of the regulation."[33]

The fundamental basis for objection to the West Virginia plan which has been articulated by HCFA has been the suggestion that the hospital funds were not "true donations". HCFA has suggested that hospitals were held hostage in the sense that the only way in which they could hope to receive payment to which they were already entitled was to "donate" to the Medically Indigent Fund, and since they themselves supplied the state's portion they were in effect receiving discounted payments.[34] One HCFA employee stated that the agency would also look very closely at any plan which seemed to involve any sort of quid pro quo between the state and providers. It is the suggestion of coercion and of quid pro quo to which HCFA ostensibly objects, and not the use of donations per se.[35]

West Virginia began the process of appealing the disallowance of the donated funds before the USDHHS grant appeals board in June of 1987. Briefs filed by HCFA's attorneys continue to maintain that the hospital funds were not "true donations" but rather short-term loans to the state Medicaid program. HCFA holds that the fact that hospitals which donated funds received claims payments in excess of their contributions on the same day that the donations were received suggests that the funds were never under full administrative control of the Medicaid agency as the regulations require. It is West Virginia's contention that the donations became eligible for FFP as soon as they were received by the state, and that there is no historical basis for interpretation of administrative control as being a function of the length of time the funds are held by the state.[36]

HCFA further contends that donations by for-profit hospitals would in any case be ineligible for match under 42 CFR Sec. 433.45 (b)(3) unless those hospitals were not also Medicaid providers. The state claims that "for-profit facilities did not receive payments on claims in excess of appropriated state funds minus the private donations."[37] The State also holds that HCFA does not have adequate authority to impose a requirement of separate accounting for private and public donations.[38]

HCFA is also proposing that the state's expenditures on claims payments should be reduced by the amount of the donations, and only this reduced amount should be considered eligible for federal match.[39] This would seem to be equivalent to holding all of the donations, regardless of whether they come from a proprietary source or not, ineligible as a source of State share. Another point on which HCFA has challenged West Virginia's plan is the issue of conditionality. HCFA maintains that the donations should be disallowed because a tacit understanding between the donating hospitals and the state existed to the effect that those hospitals would be given top priority in reimbursement. West Virginia responds that no explicit ban on conditionality is included in the regulation. Furthermore, the State contends, the old regulation allowing for training applications only of donated funds (42 CFR Sec. 432.60) did contain language specifically prohibiting conditional donations. They conclude that the choice to eliminate that language when the new regulations were drawn up indicates an intent to remove such restrictions.[40]

The USDHHS Grant Appeals Board (GAB) issued a draft decision on the case in December of 1987, which gave both parties an opportunity to comment before a final decision was rendered. In this draft the board found in favor of West Virginia, saying that the plan met all the standards currently set forth in the regulations. The board noted that HCFA seemed to be applying conditions to the regulations which do not exist, including some conditions which were expressly rejected at the time when the regulations were promulgated.[41]

Several important comments were included in the opinion. The GAB holds that the intention of the regulation permitting the donation of private funds was to allow the state to use those donations to reduce the state's share, and that the states should not have to "share" the benefit of the donations with HCFA. It is also noted that when the regulations were promulgated in 1985, HCFA rejected the inclusion of a provision that private funds could not be donated with restrictions (conditions) on their use. HCFA's characterization of the donations as short-term loans is dismissed by the observation that there is no evidence of a request for repayment by the hospitals, and that in any case there is no regulatory prohibition of the use of loans to fund the state's share.[42]

Even the use of donations from private sector providers is upheld by the preliminary opinion. The GAB accepts West Virginia's argument that because state general revenue appropriations were more than sufficient to pay for claims of private hospitals which donated funds, the state was not relying on those donations to make payments to those facilities. On this basis, the GAB holds that it can be considered that the funds donated by the private hospitals did not revert to the donors in violation of regulations.[43]

The GAB decision also discussed some of the allegations of preferential treatment of the donating hospitals. There is apparently substantial evidence that donating hospitals received reimbursement more quickly than non-donating facilities during the last quarter of 1986; in fact, payments for " clean" (fully processed) claims to donating hospitals were made within 48 hours of receipt of the donations.[44] Evidently all hospitals received all claims due them by the end of the quarter, and the GAB comments that there is no evidence that reimbursement to non-participating hospitals was delayed more than would have been the case if no donations had been made.[45]

In a similar vein, the interim reimbursement rate for hospitals was temporarily raised to 95% in November of 1986, and was reduced to 5% over the original (pre-November) rate in December. When disbursals were made in late November and again in December, very few non-donating hospitals were reimbursed.[46] The GAB draft opinion notes that although donating hospitals may have been disproportionately affected by the higher interim rate, all providers will have their paid claims adjusted either up or down when final cost reports are settled, and thus the donating hospitals have not in any sense received a "better" reimbursement rate.[47]

In concluding the draft opinion, the GAB notes that the disallowance "simply does not appear to be supported by existing regulations." The conclusion goes on to say that there is no reason why HCFA cannot attempt to change the regulations or at least issue (for the first time) official policy guidance to states to formalize the interpretation which the agency is supporting in this appeal. HCFA has in fact drafted a change in the regulations which would eliminate the use of donated funds from private sources.[48] However, it would seem that such a change would have only a minimal effect on the use of donated fund plans. In West Virginia only $3.8 million out of approximately $83 million was reimbursed to private providers.[49] Also, as is described below, HCFA has refused to approve the use of donations from exclusively public sources in Arkansas and Tennessee. It seems clear that the real issue at stake is not the use of private sector funds.

An alternative explanation for HCFA's stance has been expressed by the president of the West Virginia Hospital Association, who stated that he believes that HCFA's decision was a result of the agency's concern that "if other states did what we did, the federal government would see a significant increase in federal Medicaid matching funds."[50] Indeed, the GAB notes that "an underlying concern of the Agency's appears to be the size and scope of the state's donation program." The board points out that, as previously noted in this report, the preamble to the regulation as promulgated in 1985 specifically indicated that the donation provision was being broadened to allow states to find alternative funding sources for their Medicaid programs.[51]

The HCFA response to the draft opinion has been predictably negative, and the agency requested a hearing in March of 1988. The agency comments on the draft decision begin with a pointed discussion of the potential "catastrophic" fiscal impact which widespread use of hospital donations could have on the

Medicaid program. The HCFA comments focus on the concept that funds cannot be considered donations if they effectively revert back to the donor. Within the body of the same comments, HCFA notes that in a New Mexico case the GAB found that it was acceptable for the state to agree to require a provider (in this case, a college) to make donations towards the state's share which ultimately reverted to the provider. HCFA states that this case cannot be applied to West Virginia because the West Virginia case involves the handling of payment for services already rendered by the hospitals, rather than a prospective agreement between state and donor under which the donor agrees to accept what amounts to discounted payment.[52] While this may be a valid distinction in the West Virginia case, it is difficult to imagine how this could be used to justify the disapproval of other states' prospective donation plans.

At this writing, the GAB has not yet issued a final opinion in the case. The hearing requested by HCFA was held in March 1988, and a decision is anticipated in May 1988.

Tennessee

In March of 1987 the Tennessee General Assembly under Governor Ned McWherter passed legislation specifically authorizing the state Medicaid agency to accept donations of funds from public and private sources. The law stipulates that donations must be unconditional and unrestricted in character, and that the funds shall be under the administrative control of the agency. Contributions may not be used to reduce state general revenue funding.[53] The legislation forms the basis for a broader plan for Medicaid expansion which was successfully promoted by the Governor's office.

Under the new plan, sixteen Tennessee hospitals serving large proportions of medically indigent patients and hospitals affiliated with medical schools have agreed to donate over $19 million to the state's Medicaid program. Because Tennessee receives about 70 federal dollars for every 30 dollars the state puts up, the potential returns from such a plan are substantial.[54] The funds donated by the hospitals were combined with $3 million from the state's existing MCH program to draw federal match. As a result, Tennessee added about $70 million in 1987 to its Medicaid plan without any increase in state appropriations.[55]

The state planned to use the newly generated funds in three program areas. First, the state has adopted 1986 OBRA coverage of pregnant women and of children to age 2 up to the federal poverty level, and funds generated by the donations will be needed to produce the state's share for this coverage. Second, Medicaid coverage of inpatient hospital stays was extended from 14 to 20 days. Last, the state plans to use the proceeds to fund a program of enhanced reimbursement to hospitals which provide a disproportionate share of their services to the medically indigent.

<u>Disproportionate Share Reimbursement</u>

Since disproportionate share reimbursement has been a critical component of Tennessee's plan, an understanding of the nature and significance of this reimbursement option is important. Under the 1981 OBRA, the Medicaid Act was amended to read that state Medicaid programs must provide for payment to providers via the use of rates developed in accordance with standards "which, in the case of hospitals, take into account the situation of hospitals which serve a disproportionate number of low income patients with special needs."[56] Under this provision, states have been able to offer more generous reimbursement rates to hospitals which serve a larger number of Medicaid-eligible patients. In 1986, the U.S. Congress further clarified this provision, stating that the statute cannot be construed as authorizing HCFA or USDHHS to place any upper limits on the amount of payments states may make to disproportionate share providers.[57]

Tennessee obtained approval in June of 1987 (retroactive to October 1986) from HCFA for a state plan amendment pertaining to methods and standards for establishing payment rates for inpatient hospital services. The amendment includes a formula for providing a payment incentive (disproportionate share reimbursement) to hospitals having either over 3,000 patient days attributable to Medicaid eligible patients or a utilization ratio (percentage of patient days attributable to Medicaid eligible patients) over 14%. Hospitals which do not report having provided any charity care are not eligible for this benefit. A restriction is included which precludes the possibility of any hospital ending up with more income than it would have received if all its charity care and bad debts had actually been paid for. An incentive is also provided for hospitals which offer outpatient services to Medicaid and/or non-Medicaid indigent patients, presumably to reduce unnecessary and costly utilization of emergency room services.[58]

Because of Tennessee's generous federal match, the disproportionate share reimbursement to hospitals in the first quarter in which donations were used made it possible for every hospital but one to get more than twice its donation back in claims payments.[59] The above-mentioned incentives for hospitals which offer outpatient services are a mechanism by which the state hopes to encourage more cost-effective care for the Medicaid eligible and the medically indigent. Although no requirement for maintenance of effort by providers is included in the disproportionate share formula, the Governor's office has said that it is their hope that hospitals which benefit from enhanced reimbursement will now be able to provide more care for the medically indigent who do not qualify for Medicaid.[60]

The Omnibus Budget Reconciliation Act of 1987 instituted for the first time detailed definitions of acceptable formulas for disproportionate share reimbursement, which may override the formula now used by Tennessee.[61] Further discussion of this law is provided below; the potential impact on Tennessee's donated funds program is uncertain.

Tennessee has chosen thus far not to accept donations from for-profit hospitals. In theory proprietary entities could make donations to non-profit foundations or public interest groups which might then donate funds to the state General Fund or the Medicaid program.[62] This kind of "laundering" was used extensively under similar regulations which governed the Title XX programs, apparently with the tacit approval of federal administrators.[63] The existence of this and other such precedents strengthens the sense that the real concern of the federal administrators is the potential cost associated with increased reliance on donations rather than improper reversion of funds to donors.

The Tennessee Department of Health and Environment (TDHE) in March of 1987 submitted to HCFA a state plan amendment indicating the state's intention to use donated funds as a portion of the state's share. A request from HCFA in June of 1987 for additional information asked that the state provide a detailed description of the administrative process involved in the use of the donations. HCFA also asked for assurance that the state would continue to provide at least 40% of the total non-federal expenditures under the Medicaid program, as required by federal regulations (Tennessee's donated funds in 1987 amounted to about 2% of total Medicaid expenditures), and that localities would be protected from any diminution in services resulting from a lack of funds from local sources.[64]

Tennessee provided responses to HCFA's inquiries that same month. HCFA replied in July that the responses were insufficient for approval of the amendment, and submitted further questions aimed at identifying the precise nature of the understanding between provider-donors and the state. HCFA requested that the state respond within two weeks.[65] TDHE provided answers to the additional questions, and in October of 1987 received official notification of disapproval of the plan amendment. The basis for the rejection was that the plan amendment did not meet the generic requirements for a section 1902 State Plan amendment. This rejection did not address any substantive issues regarding the use of donated funds.[66] In November of 1987, Tennessee submitted to HCFA a petition for reconsideration of the amendment.

Some observations should be made concerning the applicability of Tennessee's experience to Texas. There are two characteristics of Tennessee's situation which have considerable impact on the donated funds-disproportionate share program. First, the hospital industry has a strong working relationship with state government. Without this relationship, the original donations plan might never have been accomplished. This atmosphere of cooperation, strengthened by the track record established with the 1987 donations, may make it possible for the state to continue to accept donations made directly to the state's general fund despite the disapproval of the state plan amendment.

Tennessee's eligibility standards and scope of services for Medicaid have traditionally been conservative. In 1985 the state set AFDC eligibility at 21.4% of federal poverty level, making Tennessee one of three states with a lower eligibility threshold than Texas.[67] However, reimbursement levels to hospitals have been high. As a result, Tennessee's Medicaid program serves a small population for which relatively few services are covered, but the amount paid to hospitals for those services which are covered is relatively high. Disproportionate share reimbursement is thus an enhancement of already generous rates and is attractive to the hospital community, which supported the Governor's plan.

Also, Tennessee's 70:30 federal matching rate guarantees hospitals a much heftier return on their donations than would be true in Texas, where the matching rate was about 55:45 for 1987, is about 57:43 for 1988, and will be increased to 59:41 in 1989.[68] It is possible, however, that disproportionate share enhancements could be made generous enough to provide an adequate incentive for hospital participation should Texas pursue such a policy.

Arkansas

Arkansas in 1987 adopted new disproportionate share provision of its Medicaid plan which incorporated a provision for the donation of funds by disproportionate share hospitals within the body of the disproportionate share formula itself.

Under this plan, hospitals averaging more than 15% total days per 12 month period as Medicaid reimbursable days would have been eligible for participation. The existing per diem reimbursement rate for an eligible hospital was to be enhanced by an amount derived from the medical portion of the Consumer Price Index.[69] The effective enhancement rate proposed was 21% over current per diem. Hospitals which choose to participate were to be given the option to donate on a quarterly basis what would be the State's portion of the enhanced reimbursement, i.e., 26% of 21% of the unenhanced per diem rate (the 1987 FFP rate for Arkansas was approximately 74%). The state plan amendment submitted by the state was, like Tennessee's, rejected by HCFA, and the State has no plans to pursue the amendment further.[70]

Arkansas has, however, implemented a program to help fund Medicaid reimbursement of nursing homes in the state. Under state law, each nursing home is assessed a licensing fee of $160 per bed. Proceeds of the fees are commingled with state general revenues, but are dedicated for use in the Medicaid nursing home program. The state has used these fees to fund a substantial increase in Medicaid reimbursement rates to the nursing homes. It is reported that legislation is being contemplated for the upcoming session of the Arkansas legislature which would establish a similar fee or tax system to supplement inpatient hospitalization reimbursement.[71]

Alabama

The state of Alabama passed legislation in August of 1987 which created the Mothers and Babies Indigent Care Trust Fund. The state hopes to attract at least $7.7 million in donations from "counties, city councils, hospitals, private foundations, individuals, etc." to fund the adoption of OBRA 86 coverage of pregnant women and children up to age one.[72] It is reported that response to the call for donations has been limited, and that the state Hospital Association has not been involved in promoting the program.[73]

The Future of Donated Funds

The Omnibus Budget Reconciliation Act of 1987 has made an impact on the status of the use of donated funds in two areas. First, Congress failed to enact an amendment which would have codified the use of voluntary contributions to state medicaid programs. Also, changes were made in the administration of disproportionate share reimbursement which may indirectly affect donated funds use by limiting the flexibility with which states may create incentives for donations through such reimbursement.

Status of Donation Regulation

The House of Representatives' version of the budget went into the reconciliation process containing a provision which would have amended section 1902(a)(2) of the Social Security Act to include "the application of private funds donated to, and subject to the unrestricted control of, the State" as an acceptable source of financial participation by the state.[74] This provision was not included in the final version of OBRA 1987 as passed onto law.

This codification would of course have precluded USDHHS from implementing a proposed regulation change. The USDHHS proposal would have restructured the applicable regulation to include an explicit description of "funds prohibited from use as the State share" which would include "funds donated from private sources, whether donated directly to the Medicaid agency or through other public agencies."[75]

As donations from the private sector were minimal in West Virginia and were not used at all in Tennessee, it would not seem that this regulatory approach would have any significant impact on the potential scope of donated funds programs. It also seems that the language prohibiting the donation of private funds through "other public agencies" would set up an unenforceable situation in which a state would be required to verify that private sector donations (made for any purpose or program) to the state's general fund are never applied to the Medicaid program.

The Reagan administration's proposal for the budget for fiscal year 1989 is reported to include a directive to USDHHS to limit hospital's donations to state Medicaid programs.[76] However, it is not yet clear how the agency intends to achieve this end. As noted, the prohibition of private donations would still allow public hospitals to donate. It would seem that USDHHS would have to prohibit donations from all sources to protect against the possibility of large scale donations. One report on the administration's plans stated that Senate Finance Committee Chairman Lloyd Bentsen opposes the elimination of donated funds as an option,[77] but it is not anticipated that the Senator from Texas will make the issue a priority in the absence of a well-defined donations plan for Texas.

Disproportionate Share Reimbursement

OBRA 1987 created for the first time specific guidelines for reimbursement of disproportionate share hospitals. Disproportionate share hospitals are defined as those with a "Medicaid inpatient utilization rate" greater than one standard deviation above the state mean, or with a "low-income utilization rate" in excess of 25%. The Medicaid inpatient utilization rate is a ratio of the number of inpatient days attributable to persons eligible on those days for Medicaid under the state plan; thus this formula will identify more hospitals as disproportionate share in states with more liberal eligibility standards, and in states which cover more days of inpatient hospitalization. The low-income utilization figure is the sum of two ratios. The first ratio expresses a hospital's Medicaid income and state and local aid as a fraction of total patient service revenues. To this figure is added the ratio of charity care charges (not including contractual disallowances for Medicaid) to total patient charges. The law does not address the thorny question of how "charity care" charges are to be delimited.[78]

Texas is one of only about a dozen states which has adopted a disproportionate share methodology, and even fewer states have actually gotten to the point of disbursing funds. TDHS made disproportionate share payments in 1987 amounting to almost $6 million. It is not clear at this point whether the law will allow states such as Texas to continue to handle disproportionate share reimbursement on a lump-sum disbursal basis, or if some sort of add-on to the disproportionate hospitals' Standard Dollar Amounts will be required, which would result in an uncapitated (and possibly substantial) increase in reimbursement costs. Texas and other states which have invested resources in developing a methodology may appeal to HCFA for grandfathered status under the 1987 law.[79]

A final item of importance in the disproportionate share provisions was the restriction requiring that a hospital must have at least two physicians with staff privileges who have agreed to provide non-emergency obstetrical services to Medicaid patients. Rural hospitals were exempted from this clause; however, hospitals are designated as "rural" according to SMSA status, and it is estimated that 150-200 small towns in Texas are classified as "urban" because of their proximity to a large urban area. This problem may result in rural hospitals being ineligible for disproportionate share reimbursement no matter how much free care they provide.[80]

Implications for Texas

Disproportionate share reimbursement may be important to any future uses of donated funds in Texas. Public hospitals, counties, or hospital districts which care to make donations to the state to help finance expansions of the Medicaid program will have a stronger incentive to do so if they can be assured that a mechanism is in place which will assure that the hospitals which serve the largest numbers of Medicaid clients are compensated for that special burden. Particularly important in Texas is the special burden of hospitals which provide a great deal of uncompensated care to undocumented aliens who are not eligible for Medicaid. The Texas Senate Select Committee on Medicaid and Family Services has established a Local Funds Subcommittee which is exploring the logistical and political feasibility of supplementing Medicaid funding with a standard local contribution or with donated funds.

The donated funds approach to Medicaid expansion could provide a politically workable infusion of funding which would benefit both hospitals and the state's poor. Even if Texas eventually chooses to pursue an across-the-board local funding system for Medicaid, a donated funds program may be a desirable temporary measure. Such a program could be quickly implemented, because participation would be voluntary and the program would not require new taxes.

Implementation of local funding, on the other hand, would be a slower process. Careful consideration will need to be given to questions of the most equitable way to tax for health care, taking into account the overall issue of tax equity and efficiency statewide. If a local funding mechanism is adopted, it should be forward-looking enough to be compatible with and to survive anticipated changes in the state taxation system whenever they may occur.

Notes

1. 42 CFR, sec. 433.33 (b),(c).

2. Telephone interview with Shelley Hagan, Wisconsin Department of Health and Social Services, Bureau of Health Care Financing, Madison, July 27, 1987.

3. TEX. REV. CIV. STAT. ANN. art. 4438f (Vernon 1976).

4. TEX. REV. CIV. STAT. ANN. art. 4438f, sec. 1.02(6), 2.011, 10.01, 12.03, 14.01 (Vernon, 1976).

5. TEX. TAX CODE ANN. sec. 26.07, subsec. (h) (Vernon 1982).

6. State Property Tax Board, "1986 County Indigent Health Care," February 1987.(Computer printout.)

7. TEX. REV. CIV. STAT. ANN. art. 4438f, sec. 10.03.

8. TEX. REV. CIV. STAT. ANN. art. 4438f, sec. 11.02.

9. Constitution of the State of Texas, Art. 9, sec 4.

10. Ibid., Art. 9., Sec. 9a.

11. State Property Tax Board, "1986 County Indigent Health Care," February 1987.(Computer printout.)

12. The Attorney General of Texas, Opinion No. JM-859, February 18, 1988.

13. 42 CFR, Ch. IV, Sec. 433.45.

14. 42 CFR, Ch. IV, Sec.433.45 (a).

15. 42CFR, Ch. IV, Sec. 433.45 (b).

16. Federal Register, Vol. 50, No. 218, , November 12, 1985, pp. 46652, 46657.

17. Ibid., p. 46652.

18. Ibid., p. 46657.

19. Ibid.

20. Federal Register, Vol. 50, No. 218, Tuesday, November 12, 1985, p. 46661.

21. Ibid., p. 46662.

22. Telephone interview with J.B. McReynolds, Deputy General Counsel, Office of the General Counsel, Texas Department of Human Resources, Austin, July 21, 1987.

23. "HCFA Challenges State's Retention of Medicaid Funds," Hospitals, (May 1987), p. 26.

24. Memorandum Opinion, U.S. District Court, Southern District of West Virginia. Civil Action No. 2:87-0333. May 12, 1987. Regina Lipscomb v. Otis Bowen.

25. Intergovernmental Health Policy Project, Major Changes in State Medicaid and Indigent Care Programs, January-December 1986, (Washington, 1986), p.70.

26. Medicare and Medicaid Guide, Commerce Clearing House, (Chicago, 1987), paragraph 14,905.

27. Ibid.

28. Telephone interview with Patty Vandergriff, reporter, Charleston Gazette, Charleston, West Virginia, August 6, 1987.

29. "HCFA Challenges State's Retention of Medicaid Funds," Hospitals, vol.61, no.10 (May 20, 1987), p. 26.

30. Memorandum Opinion, U.S. District Court, Lipscomb v. Bowen.

31. Ibid.

32. Bowen v. Lipscomb, U.S. District Court, Southern District of West Virginia, Civil Action No. 2:87-0333, Memorandum in support of Defendant's Motion to Dismiss and in Opposition to Plaintiff's Motion for Preliminary Injunction, attachments I and II.

33. Ibid.

34. Lipscomb v. Bowen, U.S. District Court, Southern District of West Virginia, Civil Action No. 2:87-0333, Memorandum in Support of Defendant's Motion to Dismiss and in Opposition to Plaintiff's Motion for Preliminary

Injunction, attachment II.

35. Telephone interview with Bill Lasowski,Director of Division of State Agency Financial Management, Health Care Financing Administration, Baltimore, June 29, 1987.

36. Telephone Interview with Frances Hughes, Assistant Attorney General, State of West Virginia, Charleston, August 10, 1987.

37. U.S. District Court, Southern District of West Virginia, Charleston Division, Civil Action no. 2:87-0333, Memorandum in Support of Plaintiff's Motion for Preliminary Injunction, April 8, 1987.

38. Ibid.

39. Ibid.

40. Ibid.

41. U.S. Department of Health and Human Services, Departmental Grant Appeals Board, Draft Decision, Board Docket Nos. 87-64 and 87-126, December, 1987, pp. 1-2.

42. U.S. Department of Health and Human Services, Departmental Grant Appeals Board, Draft Decision, Board Docket Nos. 87-64 and 87-126, December, 1987, pp. 2-3.

43. U.S. Department of Health and Human Services, Departmental Grant Appeals Board, Draft Decision, Board Docket Nos. 87-64 and 87-126, December, 1987, pp. 14-16.

44. U.S. Department of Health and Human Services, Departmental Grant Appeals Board, Agency Brief, Board Docket No. 87-64, July 1987, pp. 4-8.

45. U.S. Department of Health and Human Services, Departmental Grant Appeals Board, Draft Decision, Board Docket Nos. 87-64 and 87-126, December, 1987, p. 9.

46. U.S. Department of Health and Human Services, Departmental Grant Appeals Board, Agency Brief, Board Docket No. 87-64, July 1987, pp. 5,6.

47. U.S. Department of Health and Human Services, Departmental Grant Appeals Board, Draft Decision, Board Docket Nos. 87-64 and 87-126, December, 1987, p. 9.

48. U.S. Department of Health and Human Services, Draft Proposal for change to 42 CFR, sec. 433.45, June 15, 1987.

49. U.S. Department of Health and Human Services, Departmental Grant Appeals Board, Draft Decision, Board Docket Nos. 87-64 and 87-126, December, 1987, pp. 1, 15.

50. "HCFA Challenges State's Retention of Medicaid Funds," Hospitals, vol. 61 no.10 (May 20, 1987), p. 26.

51. U.S. Department of Health and Human Services, Departmental Grant Appeals Board, Draft Decision, Board Docket Nos. 87-64 and 87-126, December, 1987, p. 2.

52. U.S. Department of Health and Human Services, Departmental Grant Appeals Board, Agency Comments on Draft Decision, Board Docket Nos. 87-64 and 87-126, December, 1987, pp. 1,13.

53. Tennessee Code Annotated, Title 14, Chapter 23, Part 1.

54. Medicare and Medicaid Guide, Commerce Clearing House (Chicago, 1987), paragraph 14,905.

55. Cathy Tokarski, "Limits Sought on States' Use of Hospital Donations to Increase Medicaid Funds," Modern Healthcare (April 1, 1988), p. 26.

56. 42 U.S.C., sec. 1396a(a)(13)(A).

57. Omnibus Budget Reconciliation Act of 1986, P.L. 99-509, Sec. 9433.

58. State of Tennessee, State Plan Under Title XIX of the Social Security Act, Medical Assistance Program, attachment 4.19A, pp. 7,8.

59. "Shelby hospitals due state funds increase," Tennessean, March 7, 1987, sec. B, p.1.

60. "Medicaid Indigent Care Program for 1987-88," Nashville, March 5, 1987. (Flyer distributed at press conference of Governor Ned McWherter of Tennessee.)

61. Omnibus Budget Reconciliation Act of 1987, P.L. 100-203, sec. 4112.

62. Ibid.

63. Telephone interview with J.B. McReynolds, Deputy General Counsel, Office of the General Counsel, Texas Department of Human Services, Austin, August 6, 1987.

64. Letter of Response to Associate Regional Director, Division of Program Operations, HCFA Region IV, from Commissioner of Tennessee Department of Health and Environment, dated June 24, 1987.

65. U.S. Department of Health and Human Services, Health Care Financing Administration, Letter from Associate Regional Director, Division of Program Operations, HCFA Region IV, to Commissioner of Tennessee Department of Health and Environment, dated July 17, 1987.

66. U.S. Department of Health and Human Services, Letter from William L. Roper, M.D., Administrator, Health Care Financing Administration, to Commissioner James E. Word of Tennessee Department of Health and Environment, dated September 28, 1987.

67. National Health Care Campaign, Facing Facts: A Statistical Profile of Health Care in Texas, Washington, D.C., December 1986, p. HC-12.

68. Commerce Clearing House, Medicare and Medicaid Guide, March 1988, paragraph 14,905.

69. Arkansas Medical Assistance Program, General Policies and Guidelines: Hospitals; attachment 4.19-A, revised July 1, 1987, p. 5a.

70. Telephone interview with Ray Hanley, Assistant Deputy Director, Division of Economic and Medical Services, Arkansas Department of Human Services, Little Rock, December 15, 1987.

71. Telephone interview with Carol Peters, Indigent Health Care Division, Texas Department of Human Services, Austin, May 6, 1988.

72. Alabama Medicaid Agency, "Request for Proposals to Expand Medicaid Coverage to More Pregnant Women and Children," Montgomery, 1987.

73. Telephone interview with Lucille White, Alabama Foundation for Women's Health, Birmingham, December 14, 1987.

74. <u>Budget Reconciliation Act of 1987</u>, 100th Cong., 1st sess., 1987, H.R. 3545, pp. 632-633.

75. U.S. Department of Health and Human Services, Draft Proposal for change to 42 CFR, sec. 433.45, June 15, 1987.

76. Cathy Tokarski, "Limits Sought on States' Use of Hospital Donations to Increase Medicaid Funds," <u>Modern Healthcare</u> (April 1, 1988), p. 26.

77. "Congress Balks at Medicare Changes," <u>Medicine and Health</u>, vol. 42, no. 10 (March 7, 1988), p.3.

78. <u>Omnibus Budget Reconciliation Act of 1987</u>, P.L. 100-203, sec. 4112.

79. Telephone interview with Rick Peters, Director of Inpatient Reimbursement, Economic Analysis Division, Texas Department of Human Services, Austin, April 15, 1988.

80. Telephone interview with Rick Peters, Director of Inpatient Reimbursement, Economic Analysis Division, Texas Department of Human Services, Austin, May 23, 1988.

Chapter Ten
Sizing Up the Medicaid Expansion Issue

The difficulty of arriving at acceptable projections of the costs of eligibility expansions has been well illustrated by the process of the interagency work group charged with implementing H.B. 1847 for the MIHIA program. It is particularly difficult to zero in on populations eligible for Medicaid because some of the individual characteristics which determine eligibility are not information which would traditionally be collected for any reason by a health care provider. For example, when a Texas hospital provides services to a uninsured person with an income under poverty level, the facility is not likely to keep a record of the person's household structure, or of the value of his family car. More to the point, although hospitals keep track of the amount of uncompensated care they provide, information systems are not sophisticated enough to match up the free care they have provided with the detailed profiles of the patients who could not pay.

The uncertainty of projections can easily become the basis for postponing action. Fortunately, in the question of whether and how and when to expand the Medicaid program in Texas, the most compelling data may lie not in the cost and utilization projections for the various possible expansions, but instead in the fairly solid numbers describing uncompensated care and state and local indigent care programs. These latter figures may serve two purposes. First, they provide a measure of the price Texans are paying for non-participation in Medicaid. Second, they identify areas where existing resources are now being devoted to indigent health care. These resources could potentially form the basis for funding Medicaid expansions. An analysis of data on current spending and indications for alternative funding of Texas Medicaid are contained in this final chapter.

HOSPITAL DATA

When poor Texans do not qualify for any type of public medical assistance, the financial burden for their care frequently falls on the hospitals to which they resort when their medical problems demand attention. In 1986, Texas hospitals reported providing over $1.4 billion in uncompensated care to patients. Most of this free care (over 63%) is provided by public hospitals funded by city and county taxes.[1] Of course, not all of this free care could be paid for by Medicaid even under expanded eligibility; married or single adults with no children (and who are not aged, blind or disabled) will never be covered. However, the uncompensated care numbers are still good indicators of the degree to which the need for public medical assistance is not met or, more accurately, is being met by cities and counties.

The collection of hospital data has been improving steadily over the last few years, spurred on by the inclusion in the 1985 Indigent Health Care Package of new requirements for hospital data collection.[2] The 1986 Annual Survey collects information regarding the amount of total gross patient revenue and the number of admissions, discharges and patient days attributable to charity care, charity care under the Hill-Burton program, bad debt, and the various local, state and federal payor sources. Since patient demographic data are not included, we cannot determine from the data the types of patients which make up the charity care population.[3]

Table 10.1
Uncompensated Care by Ownership Type
Hospitals in Texas - 1986

	Total Hospitals	Public Hospitals	Non-Profit Hospitals	Private Hospitals
Number Reporting	458	179	135	144
Gross Patient Revenue (Millions)	$9,849.2	$2,564.3	$4,489.3	$2,795.6
Uncompensated Care* (Millions)	$1,419.0	$896.3	$368.6	$154.1
Uncompensated Care as a Percent of Gross Patient Revenue	14.4%	35%	8.2%	5.5%

*Numbers may not total due to rounding.
Uncompensated care includes both charity care and bad debt; excludes contractual adjustments.

Source: 1986 TDH/AHA/THA Annual Survey of Hospitals.

A Hospital Data Advisory Committee was authorized by Article 4438e of Texas Civil Statutes.[4] The committee is charged with both the development of reporting requirements and the interpretation and evaluation of hospital data. The committee has long-range plans to develop a hospital discharge data collection system which will also allow them to assess the impact of the use of hospital services by indigent and non-indigent patients.[5] This program when implemented should yield much useful data on the utilization patterns of indigent patients, but is not intended to include financial data.[6]

Table 10.2
Uncompensated Care by Hospital Size
Hospitals in Texas - 1986

	Total Reporting	0-50 Beds	50-99 Beds	100-299 Beds	300+ Beds
Number of Hospitals	458	145	105	143	65
Uncompensated Care as a Percent of Gross Patient Revenue	14.4%	9.0%	8.9%	8.8%	18.6%

Source: 1986 Cooperative TDH/AHA/THA Annual Survey of Hospitals.

In the 1986 Annual Survey of Hospitals (the most recent year for which data is available) conducted cooperatively by the TDH, the American Hospital Association (AHA) and the Texas Hospital Association (THA), Texas hospitals overall reported that uncompensated care equaled in amount 13.8% of gross patient revenue. Tables 10.1 and 10.2 display uncompensated care data reported by hospitals in that survey. Larger hospitals (those with 300+ beds) on the average provided uncompensated care equal to 18.6% of gross revenues. Public hospitals averaged 35.0% of gross patient revenues in uncompensated care, as compared to 5.5% for proprietary hospitals.[7] These uncompensated care estimates combine hospital estimates of "bad debt" and "charity care". Different hospitals tend to use very different definitions of charity care and bad debt, making it difficult to determine with any certainty just what uncompensated care estimates really represent. Some hospitals do not wish to have an explicit policy of providing charity care, and because of this tend to label all uncompensated care as bad debt, regardless of the income status of the client. Other hospitals only include their Hill-Burton obligation as charity care, and list all other free care under bad debt. The Hill-Burton Program was established by the Hospital Survey and Construction Act of 1946 (P.L. 79-725). Hospitals which receive financing under Hill-Burton commit to providing a certain amount of uncompensated care for a specified length of time. Because they are so obliged, "Hill-Burton uncompensated care" is usually reported separately.

Some hospitals include in charity care "contractual allowances", the difference between the rate charged to full paying patients and the reimbursement rate they actually receive from Medicaid and other third party payors, even though under Medicaid they have explicitly agreed as qualified providers to accept the contractual payments as payment in full. A more common practice is to base the dollar value of free care on the full charge price (rather than a cost-based estimate) for services rendered to non-paying patients. It can be argued that this overestimates the true cost to the hospital, and that it would be more appropriate to use the Medicaid or Medicare DRG value of services rendered to estimate uncompensated care costs. However, it is also clear from our discussion of hospital reimbursement that DRG payment may underestimate true costs in some cases, so we may want to think of the true value of uncompensated care as falling somewhere between a charge-based and a cost-based estimate.

The 1986 Annual Survey of Hospitals addressed this problem by including definitions of charity care and bad debt which hospitals were requested to follow. Because there was still no way to verify that those definitions were followed, in 1987 reporting hospitals will be asked to include a copy of their definitions of charity care and bad debt.

Hospital financial data collected by TDH is confidential, so that any data which TDH releases to the public must be handled in such a way as to hide the identity not only of individual patients but also that of individual hospitals and facilities.[8] Data on individual hospitals included in this report was provided directly by the Chief Financial Officers of those facilities to the author.

Local Resources and Indigent Care

Despite the lack of a consistent definition of uncompensated care, the numbers in Table 10.1 bring home the magnitude of the resources, unmatched by federal dollars, which are being applied to indigent health care. The total price tag of $1.4 billion is greater than the $1.1 billion in federal Medicaid funding in 1987. The $896.3 million in free care provided by public hospitals is a an even clearer indicator of the magnitude of direct local tax subsidization of indigent health care, much of which is attributable to Texas' conservative Medicaid program. If 3.5% of these tax dollars were applied to the state's share of the Medicaid program, it would cover the state's estimated 1989 costs of $30.4 million for the addition of Medicaid coverage of pregnant women and infants under age one up to 100% of poverty. A diversion of 5.5% of the $896.3 million would more than cover the estimated costs for 1989 of coverage of pregnant women and children under age 6 up to 100% of poverty, plus an enhanced services package for all those women. TDHS estimates that adoption of OBRA 1987 coverage of children under age one and pregnant women up to 185% of poverty would cost the state just over $100 million, based on utilization by over 40,000 women between 100% and 185% of poverty. Application of 11.25% of the local tax dollars now being spent on free care in public hospitals could completely finance the state's share for such an expansion.

Table 10.3 displays uncompensated care statistics from ten Texas hospitals or hospital districts which received Medicaid disproportionate share reimbursement funds in 1987. The table demonstrates the concentration of uncompensated care provided by urban public hospitals in Texas; the eight hospital districts plus Brackenridge and the two University of Texas facilities provided a total of $736,067,772 in uncompensated care in 1986, or 82% of the total amount provided by public hospitals statewide. It is interesting to note that though uncompensated care in public hospitals accounts for 35% on the average statewide (see Table 10.1), in the large urban hospital Districts (Bexar, Dallas, El Paso,

Table 10.3: IHC Resources in Selected Texas Hospitals

Hospital District	Uncompensated Care 1986;as % of Gross Patient Rev.	Hospital District Levy 1986	10% of County GRTL
Amarillo	$10,818,712 16.3%	$11,181,233	$1,063,549
Bexar County	$76,302,144 62.5%	$65,685,077	$4,387,086
Dallas County	$166,756,000 68.5%	$96,877,598	$10,196,690
El Paso County	$39,182,837* 67.4%	$15,855,562	$2,140,075
Harris County	$210,395,996 80.1%	$149,029,294	$32,645,139
Lubbock County	$26,967,701* 62.1%	$5,688,629	$802,049
Nueces County	$12,745,131 16.8%	$14,567,650	$1,770,382
Tarrant County	$48,926,779 67.9%	$40,766,965	$3,393,084
Other Hospitals			
Brackenridge (City of Austin)	$17,830,622 18.2%	**$8,495,849	$4,175,621
U.T. Health Center at Tyler	$13,369,145 45.9%	UK	$970,891

U.T. Medical Branch at Galveston	$112,772,705* 52.9%	UK	$2,105,126
Edinburg General (City)	$920,958 6.9%	**$2,136,498	$1,468,450
Mercy Regional Medical Center (NFP-Laredo)	$6,499,283 15.3%	**$381,912	$1,022,694
Totals	$743,488,013	$410,666,267	$66,140,836

Sources: 1986 Cooperative TDH/AHA/THA Annual Survey of Hospitals; State Property Tax Board.
* From FY1986 Annual Audited Financial Statements.
** TDHS Economic Analysis Division.

Lubbock, Harris and Tarrant counties) uncompensated care ranges from 62% to 80% of gross patient revenue.

One explanation for the high value of 80.1% reported by the Harris County Hospital District may be that the District only reported $935 thousand in government contractual allowances, as contrasted with $12.1 million in Dallas County, $10.2 million in Nueces County, $1.8 million in Bexar County, and $7.78 million at Mercy Medical Center in Laredo.[9] While it is not clear what the "best" method for financial reporting of these contractual allowances is, it is clear that a consistent methodology is not being applied, and this has some effect on the ranges of values of uncompensated care seen.

The hospital district levies are provided as indication of the major source of local funding for the districts.[10] In the five large urban districts, the value of uncompensated care exceeds the tax levy. In the two smaller districts, the district's levy is only slightly larger than the uncompensated care figure. Three of the non-district hospitals have recorded in this column the amount which they reported to TDHS as their annual revenue for inpatient care received from cities, counties, hospital districts and the state. These numbers are submitted by the hospitals for use in calculation of the hospitals' portion of the disproportionate share reimbursement budget. This value is supplied here as a proxy indicator of the non-federal resources supporting the uncompensated care provided by these hospitals.[11] A recent study assessed the value of City of Austin subsidies to Brackenridge at $22.1 million, however, so we can expect that these numbers will not always tell the whole story with regard to public support.[12]

The 10% of GRTL (General Revenue Tax Levy) column is provided as another measure of local resources, though the 10% obligation under the Indigent Health care act does not apply to the hospital district counties.[13] The numbers also reveal the disparity in resources between counties. Brackenridge, Edinburg and Mercy hospitals are located in counties with IHC responsibility (Travis, Hidalgo and Webb, respectively). However, Brackenridge and Edinburg General do not benefit from IHC coverage because they are city-owned. Mercy Regional is included in the sample as an example of a South Texas-Rio Grande Valley hospital. There is no one type of hospital which is truly representative of valley hospitals, but Mercy illustrates the high level of uncompensated care being provided by a relatively small facility. There is no public hospital in Laredo or in Webb County, and Mercy (a not-for-profit run by the Sisters of Mercy) provides uncompensated care with very little public support.

County Resources

The Department of Human Services maintains data on county expenditures on indigent health care for counties which wish to be eligible for state assistance and liability caps under the Indigent Health Care Act. Data collected include year-to-date expenditures by each reporting county, 10% of general revenue tax levy (GRTL), percentage of GRTL expended to date, and the amount and proportion of county payments by service type. This reporting is mandated for participants in those programs. Counties which do not report include those which are completely served by one or more hospital districts, and counties which for other reasons are unable to take advantage of the benefits under the IHC Act.

Travis County is an example of a county in the latter situation. Because the expenditures of public hospitals are not countable towards state assistance or caps, the inpatient hospital costs of Brackenridge hospital are not considered part of the county's IHC expenditures. Inpatient hospital costs typically account for the bulk of IHC costs (about 65% of county IHC expenditures statewide[14]), so Travis County is unlikely to expend 10% of its general revenue tax levy on non-hospital costs. Since reporting is only required for participants, Travis and other counties which do not anticipate qualifying for benefits opt not to report, thus adding to the difficulty of assessment of the quantity of public funding supporting indigent care in those localities. A report for March of 1988 showed 97 of 136 counties with IHC responsibilities reporting.

Table 10.4
Major Indigent Health Resources in Texas:1986

Total Hospital District Levies Reported*	$485,309,241
10% GRTL for Reporting IHC Counties**	$34,133,022
Total IHC Expenditures by Reporting Counties***	$10,894,985
10% GRTL for Counties <u>NOT</u> Reporting IHC and Without Hospital District*****	$23,462,702

Sources: *State of Texas Property Tax Board, "Hospital District Reported by CAD's in 1986," July, 1987. (Computer printout.)
** and *** Texas Department of Human Resources, "Summary, County Indigent Health Care Program, August 1987," Austin, January 20, 1988. (Monthly computer report.)
****State of Texas Property Tax Board, "1986 County Indigent Health Care," February, 1987. (Computer printout.)

The 10% of GRTL figures for counties can be thought of as the portion of a county's resources which it is obliged under the Indigent Health Care Act to make available for IHC programs. It is not, as is shown in Table 10.4, a measure of actual expenditures on indigent health care. In fact, in FY 1986-87 only three reporting counties spent 10% or more of the county GRTL. In FY 1987-88, however, it appears that counties are spending more on indigent care; as of March 31, 1988 two counties had exceeded 10% GRTL in expenditures, and five more counties were close to doing so with five months remaining in the fiscal year. Also, the total year to date expenditures on indigent care reported by counties as of March 31, 1988 was $10,595,431, which is very close to the amount shown in Table 10.4 for the entire previous fiscal year.[15]

Table 10.4 surveys county property tax resources dedicated to health care. The first item is the total amount levied by reporting hospital districts in 1986, consisting of 115 districts in 95 counties.[16] The next figure is the total of the 10% GRTL from all 102 reporting IHC counties. The next row is the actual amount spent by those counties on Indigent Health Care services in FY 86-87.[17] The last row contains a total for 10% of the GRTL of the 57 counties which did not report IHC expenditures. Some of these counties are partially served by hospital districts, and the 10% GRTL figure has been adjusted to cover only the portion of the county not served by the district.[18]

Other possible sources of funding for expansion which have been discussed are State funded programs such as University of Texas System Health Institution appropriations. The U.T. system in 1986 provided free care valued at full established prices at $325.6 million; however, the System states that only $172.7 million in costs for these services can be attributed directly to General Revenue appropriations.[19] Other State supported medical schools such as Texas Tech, Texas A & M, Baylor College of Medicine and Texas College of Osteopathic Medicine also provide funding of uncompensated or subsidized indigent care through their teaching hospitals. A good deal of the subsidized care provided by medical schools is reflected in the costs of the public hospitals they use for teaching; however, it should be recognized that there are several teaching hospitals which are not located in hospital districts. John Sealy Hospital at the University of Texas Medical Branch in Galveston, and the University of Texas Health Center at Tyler (Smith county) each provide a substantial amount of uncompensated care (see Table 10.3). Neither county contains a hospital district, and neither reports IHC expenditures to TDHS or receives IHC benefits. As such, the indigent care provided by these facilities can be considered to be largely State funded. Another anomalous situation is that of Scott and White hospital in Waco, which is not a public hospital and is used as a teaching hospital by Texas A & M.

Other programs which have had their budgets eyed for coordination with Medicaid include the TDH administered Primary Health Care, Crippled Children, and MIHIA programs. Those programs received state appropriations of $8 million, $27.1 million, and $22.2 million respectively in FY 1986-87.[20] However, the integrity of the goals of these programs may not be easily protected under Medicaid (a discussion of this problem is included in Chapter Four). The Primary Health Care program serves a population a large portion of which will remain categorically ineligible for Medicaid under the most liberal income guidelines possible. Nevertheless, it is useful to realize that there are some services being provided by each of the three programs which could conceivably be funded partly by Medicaid under an expanded program. Such a change could result in more efficient use of State funds if administrative solutions are found which protect quality of care under the looser structure of Medicaid.

A recent survey of Texas hospitals found that 46.7% of non-paying patients were admitted for pregnancy related conditions.[21] It is estimated that maternity related claims account for 30-35% of Medicaid payments in Texas, and this proportion is thought to be on the increase.[22] The gravity of the uncompensated care problem in areas which Medicaid does not address makes it all the more urgent that Texas take advantage of sources of relief which are available. This argument is apparently compelling enough to convince the Select Committee on Medicaid and Family Services to implement OBRA 1986 coverage of pregnant women and children up to 100% of poverty. This could be accomplished through reallocation of current state program dollars, a voluntary hospital contribution program, through an across-the-board local contribution, or some combination of the three. A program combining state program dollars and voluntary donations could be implemented speedily, while and across-the-board funding approach may require further study.

Closing Observations

A real understanding of the problems faced by the state of Texas in improving the Medicaid program requires at least an acquaintance with a number of discrete programs and issues. It is somewhat unfortunate that the program is so very complex. There are very few officials and policy makers with a broad understanding of the program and its intricacies, and as a result changes tend to be narrow, incremental, or both. In attempting to assess the "big picture" of Texas Medicaid this report has covered a great deal of ground, so it may be useful to reiterate some of the recurrent themes which have cropped up in this survey of Medicaid funding issues. While synthesis may not be entirely possible, it is hoped that a sense of the connections between the pieces which have been presented will be imparted.

Expansions of Texas' Medicaid program may be achieved via three different mechanisms; eligibility expansions, additional coverage of optional services, and improvements in reimbursement. A synopsis of major points in each of these areas is provided below.

Eligibility Issues

Expansion of coverage of pregnant women and of children up to age six whose incomes are below the poverty level has been recommended by the Commissioner of TDHS. The 1989 cost to the state for this expansion is projected to be $48.2 million; however, several million of this would be attributed to service enhancements mentioned below. The most recent proposal would involve the transfer of $12 million in TDH's MIHIA appropriations to TDHS, and the remainder of the 1989 costs are to be located within the TDHS budget. These state funds would be matched with approximately $66 million in new federal spending.[23]

Texas also retains the option to expand eligibility even more by covering pregnant women and children up to 185% of poverty level. Using TDHS' assumptions of a 60% participation rate in the first year and that 30% of eligible women have private insurance, an additional 28,891 births would be covered in 1989 (see Table 3.3) for women between 100%

and 185% of poverty. The additional costs to the state would be about $49.8 million, and an additional $70 million in new federal dollars would be brought into the state.

Other eligibility expansions which have been proposed for Texas include a possible increase in the income ceiling for nursing home residents from the 1987 Texas level of $658.65 per month to the maximum allowable under federal law, which is three times the SSI Federal Benefit Rate, or about $1020 in 1987. If coverage of pregnant women up to 100% of poverty is implemented, Texas will also have the option of offering greatly expanded coverage to elderly and disabled Texans with incomes up to 100% of poverty. Significant numbers of people could be covered if the state adopted a broader definition of disability. Finally, coverage of families in which the principal wage earner is unemployed could be offered.

<u>Addition of Optional Services</u>

As mentioned above, the Maternal-Child expansion now under consideration incorporates the addition of a new service type, clinic-based reimbursement. Implementation of this service, along with outreach programs, identification of high-risk pregnancies, enhanced service levels for high-risk mothers, continuous eligibility and perhaps also presumptive eligibility will require a state plan amendment and substantial administrative changes.

Service additions could also form the basis for expansions in the mental health area through the adoption of coverage of inpatient psychiatric hospitalization of the under-22 and over-65 population. Diagnostic, screening and rehabilitative services could be adopted, allowing Medicaid reimbursement of community mental health providers. Estimates of the fiscal impact of adoption of these mental health services range from a worst case of $17 million in additional annual state spending if large numbers of Medicaid recipients shift to private service providers to a best case of $54 million in net benefits to state revenues in the case of little or no utilization shift. These projections are stated as net benefits; in absolute terms, they mean that for a total state additional expenditure of $108 million, additional federal spending of $162 million could be drawn.

Reimbursement Changes

Changes in reimbursement of Medicaid providers may be critical to insuring both access to care and quality of care. We have seen that the reimbursement of community homes for the mentally retarded is at a level which providers say supports only about half of the costs of operation. Evidence has also been presented which suggests that the reimbursement methodologies for hospitals, nursing homes and physicians have resulted at times in inadequate and inequitable payment of providers.

It is in this area that further independent analysis is likely to be most useful. Future studies should address the adequacy and equity of reimbursement, but need also to encompass the question of effective expenditures; that is, what level of quality is our Medicaid spending buying? Low reimbursement may very well result in poor care for low income Texans, which can hardly be considered a cost-effective application of tax dollars.

There have been few projections made of the costs of raising reimbursement levels in any of the vendor programs. But there are clearly costs associated with low reimbursement, such as the $35 million state funded PPP program to support ICF-MRs. Rural hospitals face potential losses of disproportionate share reimbursement because they cannot attract the two Medicaid obstetricians required under federal formula, largely because physician reimbursement in obstetrics is inadequate. And the demise of rural hospitals, possibly hastened by methodologies which discriminate against rural providers, represents a serious problem in this large, still significantly rural state.

Funding

As was illustrated in earlier sections of this chapter, there are enormous amounts of money being spent on indigent health care in Texas outside the Medicaid program. Many improvements in the delivery of health services to poor Texans could be achieved through reallocation of these existing resources, rather than creation of new revenues. Some redistribution of state program funds, such as the transfer from MIHIA funds proposed for the MCH expansions in Medicaid, are both logical and compatible with policy goals. The caveat should be added that such transfers should be accompanied by careful consideration of approaches to Medicaid which can guarantee that quality of care and cost effective delivery of care will be maintained under Medicaid. It must be recognized that under existing federal guidelines, many poor Texans will not be eligible for Medicaid even under the most generous program possible.

It would therefore be precipitous for lawmakers to gut state programs to fund Medicaid expansion, no matter how desirable such an expansion may be.

If handled properly, it would appear that a combination of maternal and child expansions up to 185% of poverty and the MHMR expansions outlined above could bring $298 million in new federal spending (66 + 70 + 162) to Texas for a cost to the state of $206 million (48.2 + 49.8 + 108). The result would be the extension of services to many more Texans with a net savings of $92 million.

At this writing, there appears to be some momentum among public providers with substantial numbers of low income deliveries to join together and commit funds from their various jurisdictions towards funding the MCH Medicaid expansions. Such an effort will be laudable if it can convince policy makers to implement the new eligibility standards. The fact that this approach to funding has such appeal points up several fundamental characteristics of the health care delivery network in Texas which act as underlying barriers to change. First, there is a need for far greater integration of service delivery in the interest both of cost effective care and quality care. However, movement in this direction is hampered by an understandable reflexive turf protection which occurs at the state agency level all the way down to the smallest local service providers. Strong leadership and sustained and committed efforts will be required to break through this resistance.

Integration needs to take place not only in the delivery of health care services, but also in the funding of those services. Localization of indigent health care funding cuts Texas off from 60% federally funded Medicaid dollars, which is a sort of home rule which beleaguered cities can ill afford. Local responsibility for health care should be made consistent across the state, and that responsibility could easily include funding some portion of Medicaid. Finally, the fact that the state has had to go hunting in local jurisdictions for Medicaid funding reminds us again of the inadequacy of our state revenue generation system. With funding of public schools, prisons, mental hospitals, and schools for the mentally retarded all being judged inadequate in the courts, the time is drawing near when Texas will have to find a new way to fund these programs which are so critical to quality of life and economic well being in the state.

Notes

1. Texas Department of Health, Indigent Health Care Programs, Annual Report, 1988.(Undated pre-publication draft.)

2. TEX. REV. CIV. STAT. ANN. art. 4438e (Vernon 1976).

3. American Hospital Association-Texas Department of Health-Texas Hospital Association, "1986 Annual Survey of Hospitals," Austin, 1986.(Survey instrument.)

4. TEX. REV. CIV. STAT. ANN. art. 4438e, Sec. 8 (Vernon, 1976).

5. Texas Department of Health, Request for Proposal for Hospital Data Advisory Committee, Spring, 1987.(Developed by Bureau of State Health Planning and Resource Development {name has since changed to Bureau of State Health Data and Policy Analysis} for project which was deferred.)

6. Telephone interview with Charlene Harris, Supervisor of Data Collection and Distribution Section, Data Management Division, Bureau of State Health Data and Policy Analysis, Texas Department of Health, Austin, July 24, 1987.

7. Texas Department of Health, Indigent Health Care Programs, Annual Report, 1988.(Undated pre-publication draft.)

8. TEX. REV. CIT. STAT. ANN. art. 4438e, sec. 7, (Vernon 1976).

9. American Hospital Association, TDH/AHA/THA 1986 Annual Survey of Hospitals, pp. 13, 27; for Harris, Dallas, Bexar, and Nueces County Hospital Districts and Mercy Regional Medical Center, Laredo. (Provided by individual hospitals.)

10. State of Texas Property Tax Board, "Hospital District Reported by CAD's in 1986," July, 1987. (Computer printout.)

11. Texas Department of Human Services, Economic Analysis Division, "Calculation of Disproportionate Share Ratio by Hospital," October, 1987. (Computer printout.)

12. Mary Hartman and Tommy Tompkins, Strategic Plan for Brackenridge Hospital (Fall 1987), p. 34. (Report Prepared for the Graduate School of Business, University of texas at Austin.)

13. State of Texas Property Tax Board, "1986 County Indigent Health Care," February, 1987. (Computer printout.)

14. Texas Department of Human Resources, "Summary, County Indigent Health Care Program, August 1987," Austin, January 20, 1988. (Monthly computer report.)

15. Texas Department of Human Resources, "Summary, County Indigent Health Care Program, March 1988," Austin, April 29, 1988. (Monthly computer report.)

16. State of Texas Property Tax Board, "Hospital District Reported by CAD's in 1986," July, 1987. (Computer printout.)

17. Texas Department of Human Resources, "Summary, County Indigent Health Care Program, August 1987," Austin, January 20, 1988. (Monthly computer report.)

18. State of Texas Property Tax Board, "1986 County Indigent Health Care," February, 1987. (Computer printout.)

19. University of Texas System, "U.T. System Health Institutions: Value of Free Care Provided - FY86," Austin, March 13, 1987.(Photocopied flyer.)

20. Texas Department of Health, Annual Report: Indigent Health Care Programs (Austin, February 1987), pp. 5, 29.

21. Texas Department of Health, Indigent Health Care Programs, Annual Report, February 1, 1987, p. 31.

22. Telephone interview with Rick Peters, Director of Inpatient Reimbursement Section, Texas Department of Human Services, Austin, August 17, 1987.

23. Texas Department of Human Services, "Service Enhancements in Response to the Select Committee on Medicaid and Family Services," Austin (May 4, 1988), p.5. (Agenda Item No. 8, Texas Board of Human Services meeting of May 19, 1988.)

Bibliography

Alabama Medicaid Agency. "Request for Proposals to Expand Medicaid Coverage to More Pregnant Women and Children," Montgomery, 1987.

American Hospital Association, Texas Department of Health, Texas Hospital Association. "1986 Annual Survey of Hospitals," Austin, 1986.(Survey instrument.)

Anderson, Ron J., M.D. "The Flip Side of Health Care Expenditures in Texas," Texas Medicine, vol. 84 (February 1988), p.7.

Anderson, Ron. J. President and Chief Executive Officer, Parkland Memorial Hospital (Dallas, Texas). Testimony before Lieutenant Governor's Select Committee on Medicaid and Family Services, Texas Legislature, Austin, February 17, 1988, (Written copy of testimony presented.)

Arkansas Medical Assistance Program. General Policies and Guidelines: Hospitals; attachment 4.19-A, revised July 1, 1987.

The Attorney General of Texas. Opinion No. JM-859, February 18, 1988.

Austin American-Statesman. "Funds Cut to Homes for the Retarded," April 6, 1988.

Austin American-Statesman. "Homes May Be Told to Return Medicaid Funds," March 30, 1988.

Austin American-Statesman. "State Inquiry Targets Homes for the Retarded," March 18, 1988.

Bailey, Charles, King Hillier and Dick Kreiter. Texas Hospital Association TAG. "Memorandum Regarding Appeal Rules-Medicaid Prospective System," October 2, 1987.

Bellamy, Gail, Stephen Svadlenak, Richard Peters and Donald R. Kelley. "Medicaid DRG System Being Improved for Texas Children," Texas Hospitals, Vol. 43 no. 1, June 1987, p. 14.

Buescher, Paul A. "Source of Prenatal Care and Infant Birthweight: the Case of a North Carolina County," SCHS Studies, no. 39 (March 1986).

Chapman, Jerome. Executive Director, Texas Health Care Association. "From Old Folks Homes to the Medical Model," 1987.(adapted from speech to first annual Gerontological Conference of the University of Texas Health Science Center at Houston.)

Chapman, Jerome. Executive Director of Texas Health Care Association. Testimony before Texas House of Representative Budget and Oversight of Human Services Committee, February 25, 1987.

Commerce Clearing House. Medicare and Medicaid Guide, (Chicago, 1987).

Congressional Budget Office. "Medicaid Medical Vendor Payments by Maintenance Assistance Status of Recipient, Fiscal Year 1985," May 1, 1986. (Computer printout.)

Conlon, Richard Thomas. The Medical Cost of AIDS. (Professional Report, Lyndon B. Johnson School of Public Affairs, University of Texas at Austin, December 1987.)

El Paso Times. "Proposal Would Make More Mothers-To-Be Eligible for Medicaid," April 8, 1988.

Erdman, Karen and Sidney M. Wolfe, M.D. Poor Health Care for Poor Americans (Washington, D.C.: Public Citizen Health Research Group, 1988).

Farr, George. President and Chief Executive Officer, Children's Medical Center of Dallas. Testimony before Select Committee on Medicaid and Family Services, Austin, February 11, 1988. (Written copy of testimony presented.)

Federal Register. Vol. 50, No. 218, Tuesday, November 12, 1985, p. 46661.

Fraser, Irene. Medicaid Options: State Opportunities and Strategies for Expanding Eligibility, (Chicago: American Hospital Association, 1987.)

Fredrickson, Barry. Assistant Commissioner of Client Services Branch, Texas Department of Human Services. Letter to Texas Health Care Association, April 9, 1987.

Fritz, Randy. "A Physician Survey of Texas' Liability Crisis: Impacts on Indigent Patient Care." (Summary reproduced by Texas Medical Association of a study done at LBJ School of Public Affairs, University of Texas at Austin, 1985.)

Garland, Susan B. and Gail DeGeorge. "A Welfare Mother's Battle to Clean Up the Medicaid Mess," Business Week, no. 3031 (December 21, 1987), p. 42.

Gibbs, C.E. Member MIHIA Advisory Committee. Testimony before Select Committee on Medicaid and Family Services, State Senate of Texas, February 11, 1988.

Gornick, M., et.al. "Twenty Years of Medicare and Medicaid: Covered Populations, Use of benefits, and Program expenditures," Health Care Financing Review, 1985 annual supplement.

Hartman, Mary and Tommy Tompkins. Strategic Plan for Brackenridge Hospital. Austin, Fall 1987.

(Report prepared for the Graduate School of Business, University of Texas at Austin.)

Healthcare Financial Management Association. Long-Term Care: Challenges and Opportunities (Oak Brook, Illinois, 1985).

Hospitals. "HCFA Challenges State's Retention of Medicaid Funds," (May 1987).

Intergovernmental Health Policy Project. Major Changes in State Medicaid and Indigent Care Programs, January-December 1986, (Washington, 1986).

Johnson, Richard. Texas Association of Private Providers. Testimony before Texas Board of Human Services (agenda item no. 5), Austin, December 17, 1987.

Johnston, Marlin W. Commissioner, Texas Department of Human Services. Recommendation to Texas Board of Human Services, "AZT Coverage in the Vendor Drug Program," agenda item no. 8 (December 1, 1987).

Jones, Burnham B. Senior Vice President, Finance,Texas Hospital Association. "Memorandum: Texas Medicaid PPS Report 1," April 22, 1987.

Jones, Donna B. "Rural Hospitals, Changing with the Times," Texas Medicine, vol. 84 (February 1988), p.58.

Lennie, J.A. "Low-Birth-Weight Rate Reduced by the Obstetrical Access Project," Health Care Financing Review, no. 8 (1987), pp. 83-86.

Medicine and Health. "Congress Balks at Medicare Changes," vol. 42, no. 10 (March 7, 1988).

National Governors' Association State Medicaid Information Center. "Annualized Medicaid Eligibility Thresholds - AFDC, Medically Needy, SSI - As Percent of Poverty," December 1986. (Chart.)

National Health Care Campaign. Facing Facts: A Statistical Profile of Health Care in Texas, Washington, D.C., December, 1986.

National Heritage Insurance Company. Letters to Medicaid providers and attached "Summary: Texas-based DRG Payment System," May 21, 1986.

National Heritage Insurance Company. "Texas-based Diagnosis Group Payment System, Revised April 1, 1987 (Revision II)," Austin, April 1987.

North Carolina Division of Medical Assistance. Operational Manual for Maternity Care Coordinator, Raleigh, n.d.

The Number News. "Estimates of U.S. Resident Population by State: 1980, 1984 and 1985," February 1986, reproduced by Texas Department of Human Services.

Peters, Rick. Director of Inpatient Reimbursement, Economic Analysis Division. Letter to Medicaid providers regarding SDA methodology and attached sheet, "Definitions and Calculations Used in Attachment A," dated September 23, 1987.

Rosenbaum, Sara. "Medicaid Eligibility for Pregnant Women: Reforms Contained in the Sixth Omnibus Budget Reconciliation Act," (Children's Defense Fund, Washington, D.C., April 1987).

Rosenbaum, Sara. Children's Defense Fund. "Opportunities for Expanding the Scope of Indigent Health Activities in Texas That Can Be Financed as Medicaid Expenditures", December 3, 1986. (Memorandum.)

State Property Tax Board of Texas. "Hospital Districts Reported by CAD's in 1986," July, 1987. (Computer printout.)

State Property Tax Board of Texas. "1986 County Indigent Health Care," February 1987.(Computer printout.)

State of Tennessee. Medical Assistance Program, <u>State Plan Under Title XIX of the Social Security Act</u>, attachment 4.19(A), pp. 7,8.

Tax Foundation, "Federal Grants No Bargain in FY85 for 20 States Whose Average Tax `Cost' Per Aid

Dollar Was $1.19," Washington, D.C., May 1986. (News Release.)

Tennessee Department of Health and Environment. Letter of Response to Associate Regional Director, Division of Program Operations, HCFA Region I. Dated June 24, 1987.

Tennessee Department of Health and Environment. "Medicaid Indigent Care Program for 1987-88," Nashville, March 5, 1987. (Flyer distributed at press conference of Governor Ned McWherter of Tennessee.)

Tennessean. "Shelby Hospitals Due State Funds Increase," March 7, 1987.

Texas A & M University. Public Policy Resources Laboratory. "Texas OB Survey: Determining the Need for Maternity Services in Texas - County Projections," (Submitted to Texas Department of Health, May 22, 1987).

Texas Department of Health. Indigent Health Care Programs, Annual Report, 1988. (Pre-publication draft.)

Texas Department of Health. Indigent Health Care Programs, Annual Report, February 1, 1987.

Texas Department of Health. MIHIA Contracts, December 12, 1987. (Computer Printout.)

Texas Department of Health. Request for Proposal for Hospital Data Advisory Committee, Spring, 1987.(Developed by Bureau of State Health Planning and Resource Development {name has since changed to Bureau of State Health Data and Policy Analysis} for project which was deferred.)

Texas Department of Health and Texas Department of Human Services. "Maternal and Infant Health Care for Low-Income Texans: Memorandum of Understanding," Austin (March 1988). (Final Report to Commissioners.)

Texas Department of Human Services. "AFDC-Related Medicaid Programs," January 1986. (Memorandum prepared for U.S. Congressman J.J. Pickle.)

Texas Department of Human Services. Agenda Item no. 4, Meeting of Texas Board of Human Services, December 17, 1987.

Texas Department of Human Services. "Calculation of Disproportionate Share Ratio by Hospital," October, 1987. (Computer printout.)

Texas Department of Human Services. "Comparison of Resource Requirements." Austin, February 1988. (Materials prepared for Select Committee on Medicaid and Family Services.)

Texas Department of Human Services. Feasibility Study-Drug Manufacturers Rebate Program: Why a Manufacturer's Rebate? (Austin, February 1987).

Texas Department of Human Services. "Federal Legislation Briefing: Select Committee on Medicaid and Family Services," Austin (December 4, 1987), Part IV, p.6. (Photocopied for distribution to Select Committee on Medicaid and Family Services.)

Texas Department of Human Services. Fiscal Year 1987: Year-end Budget Report, Austin (December 17, 1987).

Texas Department of Human Services. Form HCFA-2082, "Statistical Report on Medical Care: Eligibles, Recipients, Payments and Services," for fiscal year ending September 30, 1986.

Texas Department of Human Services. Legislative Appropriations Request FY 1988-89, July 7, 1986.

Texas Department of Human Services. "Medicaid Eligibility in Texas (Title XIX)," January 1, 1987. (photocopied guidelines prepared for Rep. Jake Pickle.)

Texas Department of Human Services. "Nursing Home Case Mix Demonstration Project," October 21, 1987, (draft) as cited in briefing paper prepared by Linda Logan.

Texas Department of Human Services. "Reimbursement Methodology for the Pharmacy Dispensing Fee," Austin, January 1988. (Draft of proposed methodology.)

Texas Department of Human Services. "Reimbursement Rates for FY 1988 for Community Based Intermediate Care Facilities for the Mentally Retarded." Austin (December 17, 1987), p.2. (Agenda Item No. 5, Texas Board of Human Services meeting of same date.)

Texas Department of Human Services. "Service Enhancements in Response to the Select Committee on Medicaid and Family Services." Austin (May 4, 1988), p.5. (Agenda Item No. 8, Texas Board of Human Services meeting of May 19, 1988.)

Texas Department of Human Services. <u>State Plan Under Title XIX of the Social Security Act Medical Assistance Program</u>, attachment 3.1 (A) and attachment to same.

Texas Department of Human Services. "States' Population Compared to Federal Medicaid Expenditures," June, 1986. (Background information for presentation by Director of indigent health care program.)

Texas Department of Human Resources. "Summary, County

Indigent Health Care Program," Austin, August 1987 and March 1988. (Monthly computer report.)

Texas Department of Human Services. Budget and Data Analysis Division. "Number of Births to Women with Income Below 100% of Poverty Not Receiving Medicaid or MIHIA Services," February 17, 1988. (Handouts presented to select Committee on Medicaid and Family Services.)

Texas Department of Human Services. Budget and Data Analysis Division. "Number of Births to Women with Income Below 185% of Poverty Not Receiving Medicaid or MIHIA Services," February 17, 1988. (Handouts presented to select Committee on Medicaid and Family Services.)

Texas Department of Human Services. Budget and Data Analysis Division. Presentation by Bryan Packard to Select Committee on Medicaid and Family Services, March 30, 1988.

Texas Department of Human Services. Budget and Planning Division. "1985 Special Texas Census: Summary of Selected Findings," Austin, October 15, 1986. (Photocopied.)

Texas Department of Human Services and Texas Department of Mental Health and Mental Retardation. Extending Medicaid to Cover Mental Health Services: A Report to the Lieutenant Governor, (Austin, March 15, 1985).

Texas Department of Mental Health and Mental Retardation. "Medicaid Optional Service: Inpatient Psychiatric Under 22," (Draft of report by Touche Ross, Austin, 1987).

Texas Department of Mental Health and Mental Retardation. "Medicaid Optional Services: Institutes for Mental Diseases for Patients Over 65," (Draft of report by Touche Ross, Austin, 1987).

Texas Department of Mental Health and Mental Retardation. "Option: Diagnostic,Screening and Rehabilitation," (Draft of report by Touche Ross, Austin, 1987).

Texas Health Care Association. Executive Summary of study of Nursing Home Reimbursement Methodology, March 1987. (Copy of material provided to 70th Texas legislature.)

Texas Hospital Association. "Memorandum: Update - Texas Medicaid Prospective Payment System," August 14, 1987.

Texas Hospital Association. "Technical Advisory Group-Report Number 1: Projected Losses of Texas Medicaid PPS," 1986.

Texas Hospital Association. "Technical Advisory Group, Report Number 3, Texas Medicaid PPS: Status Report of All Activities," October 13, 1986.

Texas Hospital Association. "Testimony of the THA: TDHS Public Hearing, Texas Medicaid PPS," December 3, 1986. (Draft.)

Texas Legislature. Senate Select Committee on Medicaid and Family Services. "Draft Recommendations," (presented in Austin at March 30, 1988 meeting).

Texas Long-Term Care Coordinating Council for the Elderly. "Recommendations to the 70th Legislature," December 1986.

Texas Medical Association. "Documenting the Crisis: A Survey of Texas' Primary Care Physicians." (Enclosure in packet of information provided to Select Committee on Medicaid and Family Services), Austin, February 11, 1988.

Texas Medical Association. "Professional Liability Premiums (TMLT) 10/87: Maximum Rates after 4 Years Claims." (Figures provided by to Dr. Donald Kelley, deputy Commissioner for Health Care Services, Texas Department of Human Services, October 26, 1987.)

Texas Medical Association. "Report of Reference Committee on Socioeconomics," November 1987.

Texas Medical Association Ad Hoc Committee on Physician Reimbursement. "Report to the Texas Medical Association Executive Board," April 5, 1981.

Texas Pharmaceutical Association. "Pharmacy Management: Third Party Programs," item 58, adopted 1987. (Official adopted stands of the TPA.)

Texas State Board of Insurance. The Long Term Care Dilemma: What Can Be Done About It?" January 1987. (Report to the 70th Texas Legislature.)

Tokarski, Cathy. "Limits Sought on States' Use of Hospital Donations to Increase Medicaid Funds," Modern Healthcare (April 1, 1988), p. 26.

Tonn, Larry L. Texas Department of Human Services, "Calculation of the Economic Index Factor," (Photocopied report prepared for informational use), August 20, 1981.

University of South Carolina School of Public Health. Department of Health Administration, Department of Epidemiology and Biostatistics. Evaluation of the South Carolina Medicaid High Risk Channeling Project, (Columbia, October 1987).

University of Texas System. Office of Governmental Relations. "U.T. System Health Institutions: Value of Free Care Provided - FY86," Austin, March 13, 1987.(Photocopied flyer.)

U.S. Bureau of the Census. "Resident Population by Age and State: 1985," Statistical Abstract of the United States: 1987, 107th edition, Washington, D.C., 1986.

U.S. Congress. House Committee on the Budget. Budget Reconciliation Act of 1987, 100th Cong., 1st sess., December 22, 1987, H.R. 3545, pp. 632-633.

U.S. Congress. House Committee on the Budget. The Omnibus Budget Reconciliation Act of 1986. 99th Cong., 2d sess., H.R. 5300, October 17, 1986, pp. 184-211. (Subtitle E - Medicaid and Maternal and Child Health, 391-415.)

U.S. Congress. House Committee on Ways and Means. Background Material and Data on Programs Within the Jurisdiction of the Committee on Ways and Means, 99th Cong., 2nd sess., March 3, 1986, p. 468.

U.S. Congress. Select Committee on Aging. Medicare and Medicaid Reform: Protecting the Aged and Indigent in Texas, 99th Cong., 1st sess., 1985, p. 44.

U.S. Department of Health and Human Services. Draft Proposal for change to 42 CFR, sec. 433.45, June 15, 1987.

U.S. Department of Health and Human Services. "Medicaid Assistance Payments - Federal Share, FFY 1985," Medicaid Financial Management Report, 1986, reproduced by Texas Department of Human Services.

U.S. Department of Health and Human Services. Program Memorandum, Medicaid State Agencies, HCFA-Pub. 17, Transmittal No. 86-15, August 1986.

U.S. Department of Health and Human Services. Departmental Grant Appeals Board, Agency Brief, Board Docket No. 87-64, July 1987.

U.S. Department of Health and Human Services. Departmental Grant Appeals Board, Draft Decision, Board Docket Nos. 87-64 and 87-126, December, 1987.

U.S. Department of Health and Human Services. Departmental Grant Appeals Board, Agency Comments on Draft Decision, Board Docket Nos. 87-64 and 87-126, December, 1987.

U.S. Department of Health and Human Services. Health Care Financing Administration. Letter from Associate Regional Director, Division of Program Operations, HCFA Region IV, to Commissioner of Tennessee Department of Health and Environment, dated July 17, 1987.

U.S. Department of Health and Human Services. Health Care Financing Administration. Letter from William L. Roper, M.D., Administrator, to Commissioner James E. Word of Tennessee Department of Health and Environment, dated September 28, 1987.

U.S. District Court. Southern District of West Virginia, Charleston Division. Civil Action no. 2:87-0333, Lipscomb v. Bowen. Memorandum in Support of Plaintiff's Motion for Preliminary Injunction, April 8, 1987.

U.S. District Court. Southern District of West Virginia. Civil Action No. 2:87-0333, Lipscomb v. Bowen. Memorandum in support of Defendant's Motion to Dismiss and in Opposition to Plaintiff's Motion for Preliminary Injunction, attachments I and II.

U.S. District Court. Southern District of West Virginia. Civil Action No. 2:87-0333, Lipscomb v. Bowen. Memorandum Opinion, May 12, 1987.

Vanderpool, David, M.D. President, Texas Medical Association, Cover letter to information packet for Select Committee on Medicaid and Family Services, February 11, 1988.

Wayne State University School of Medicine, Department of Pediatrics. "Average Days in Hospital for Different Birthweight Groups (survivors and non-survivors)," Detroit, n.d. (Photocopied handout.)

Interviews

Alexander, Barbara, R.N., M.N. Department Head, Department of Obstetrics and Gynecology- High

Risk Care, South Carolina Health and Human Services Financing Commission, Columbus, South Carolina. Telephone interview, July 23, 1987.

Bellamy, Gail. Health Policy Analyst, Division of Future Policy Alternatives, Texas Department of Human Services, Austin. Telephone interviews December 2, 1987 and May 24, 1988.

Cook, David. Director of Budgeting, Services to Aged and Disabled, Texas Department of Human Services. Telephone interviews November 20 and 24, 1987.

Cardenas, Doreen. Provider Enrollment, National Heritage Insurance Company, Austin. Telephone interview March 22, 1988.

Crawford, Dorothy. Executive Assistant for Government Relations, Texas Health Care Association, Austin. Interview October 1, 1987.

Gladden, Pat. Director of Policy and Audit, Vendor Drug Program, Texas Department of Human Services, Austin. Telephone interview February 19, 1988.

Hagan, Shelley. Wisconsin Department of Health and Social Services, Bureau of Health Care Financing, Madison. Telephone interview July 27, 1987.

Hanley, Ray. Assistant Deputy Director, Division of Economic and Medical Services, Arkansas

Department of Human Services, Little Rock. Telephone interview December 15, 1987.

Harris, Charlene. Supervisor of Data Collection and Distribution Section, Data Management Division, Bureau of State Health Data and Policy Analysis, Texas Department of Health, Austin. Telephone interview July 24, 1987.

Hughes, Frances. Assistant Attorney General, State of West Virginia, Charleston. Telephone Interview August 10, 1987.

Kamis, Ken. Director of Division of Primary Care, South Carolina Health and Human Services Financing Commission, Columbus, South Carolina. Telephone interview July 27, 1987.

Kirk, Ken, Phd. Associate Dean, School of Pharmacy, University of Texas at Austin, Austin. Interview January 14, 1988.

Hudson, Lynn, R.N., N.P. Nurse Consultant, Bureau of Maternal and Child Health, Texas Department of Health, Austin. Interview July 29, 1987.

Lasowski, Bill. Director of Division of State Agency Financial Management, Health Care Financing Administration, Baltimore. Telephone interview June 29, 1987.

McClure, Spencer. Executive Director, Texas Council of

Community MHMR Centers, Austin. Telephone interview December 14, 1987.

McReynolds, J.B. Deputy General Counsel, Office of the General Counsel, Texas Department of Human Resources, Austin. Telephone interview July 21, 1987.

Peters, Carol. Indigent Health Care Division, Texas Department of Human Services, Austin. Telephone interview May 6, 1988.

Peters, Rick. Director Inpatient Reimbursement Division, Economic Analysis Division, Texas Department of Human Services, Austin. Interview October 6, 1987; Telephone interviews August 17, 1987, November 30, 1987, April 15, 1988, and May 23, 1988.

Schmid, Ernest. Director Indigent Health Care Program, Texas Department of Human Services, Austin. Interview November 11, 1988.

Vandergriff, Patty. Reporter, Charleston Gazette, Charleston, West Virginia. Telephone interview August 6, 1987.

White, Lucille. Alabama Foundation for Women's Health, Birmingham. Telephone interview December 14, 1987.

Williams, Dennis. Assistant Director of Medical Policy and Utilization Control, Division of Medical

Assistance, North Carolina Department of Human Services, Raleigh. Telephone interview July 22, 1987.

Wolff, Ann. Chief of Maternal and Child Health section, North Carolina Department of Human Services, Raleigh. Telephone interview July 21, 1987.